100 Questions & Answers About Overactive Bladder and Urinary Incontinence

Pamela Ellsworth, MD

Division of Urology, University of Massachusetts Memorial Healthcare

David A. Gordon, MD, FACS

University of Maryland and Chesapeake Urology Center for Continence & Pelvic Floor Disorders

JONES AND BARTLETT PUBLISHERS
Sudbury, Massachusetts
BOSTON   TORONTO   LONDON   SINGAPORE

World Headquarters

Jones and Bartlett
Publishers
40 Tall Pine Drive
Sudbury, MA 01776
info@jbpub.com
www.jbpub.com

Jones and Bartlett
Publishers Canada
2406 Nikanna Road
Mississauga, ON L5C
2W6
CANADA

Jones and Bartlett
Publishers International
Barb House, Barb
Mews
London W6 7PA
UK

Jones and Bartlett's books and products are available through most bookstores and online booksellers. To contact Jones and Bartlett Publishers directly, call 800-832-0034, fax 978-443-8000, or visit our website *www.jbpub.com.*

Substantial discounts on bulk quantities of Jones and Bartlett's publications are available to corporations, professional associations, and other qualified organizations. For details and specific discount information, contact the special sales department at Jones and Bartlett via the above contact information or send an email to specialsales@jbpub.com.

Library of Congress Cataloging-in-Publication Data
Ellsworth, Pamela.
  100 questions and answers about overactive bladder and urinary incontinence / Pamela Ellsworth, David A. Gordon.
    p. cm.
  ISBN 0-7637-4546-4
  1. Urinary incontinence--Popular works. I. Title: One hundred questions and answers about overactive bladder and urinary incontinence. II. Gordon, David A. III. Title.
  RC921.I5E43 2005
  616.6'2--dc22

2005005145

Production Credits
Executive Publisher: Christopher Davis
Special Projects Editor: Elizabeth Platt
Production Director: Amy Rose
Associate Production Editor: Renée Sekerak
Editorial Assistant: Kathy Richardson
Manufacturing Buyer: Therese Bräuer
Marketing Manager: Matthew Payne
Cover Design: Colleen Halloran
Cover Images shown clockwise: © Creatas/PictureQuest; Anne Rippy/
  PictureQuest; BenareStock/Creatas/PictureQuest
Printing and Binding: Malloy, Inc.
Cover Printing: Malloy, Inc.

Printed in the United States of America
09 08 07 06 05   10 9 8 7 6 5 4 3 2 1

Contents

Overactive bladder (OAB) and urinary incontinence affect over 30 million male and female Americans. The risk of developing overactive bladder increases with age in both males and females. These conditions, overactive bladder and urinary incontinence, are associated with a significant negative impact on quality of life and such medical problems as urinary tract infections, skin irritation and in the elderly an increased risk of falls and fractures. Urinary incontinence is responsible for nearly 50 percent of nursing home admissions. There is a huge economic impact of these conditions also. Continence supplies, such as diapers and pads, are only a portion of the healthcare dollars spent on these conditions.

YET, despite the high prevalence, the significant effects on quality of life, the associated medical morbidities and the financial impact of these conditions, they remain largely undiagnosed and untreated. WHY is this the case? Unfortunately, there are several barriers to the identification and treatment of these conditions on both the part of the patient and the physician. Sufferers of these conditions may believe that (1) the condition(s) is an inevitable part of aging, an incorrect assumption, (2) the condition is too embarrassing to discuss with the physician, (3) the symptoms are "minor" compared to those of their friends/family with "life-threatening" illnesses and thus trivialize their own problems, and (4) there is no effective treatment, again an incorrect assumption. Some individuals may bring the subject up with their doctors but receive no evaluation or treatment. Physicians currently have no validated screening tools to assist them in the evaluation of these conditions. In addition, physicians will often wait for the patient to bring up the problem, which, as stated, is often difficult for the patient to do. Once the situation is noted, there is often a lack of evaluation and treatment. Lastly, the management of overactive bladder and urinary incontinence is continually evolving and physicians need to be aware of the newer therapies in order to best counsel patients.

Many of these limitations to the evaluation and management of overactive bladder and urinary incontinence are a result of the lack of knowledge about these conditions. It is our sincere hope that this book provides knowledge to empower OAB and urinary incontinence sufferers to seek help and to be actively involved in their management plan so that their quality of life and medical health may be improved. If we can touch the lives of even a few OAB and urinary incontinence sufferers, we will have achieved our goal. Read on and find out how you can take control of a problem(s) that has taken control of your life.

PART ONE

The Basics

What is the bladder and what does it do?

What are normal voiding habits?

What problems can occur with bladder function?

More ...

1. What is the bladder and what does it do?

The bladder is a hollow organ shaped like a sphere that is specially designed to accomplish two tasks. It stores urine at low pressures, and when the bladder is full it empties urine. For the bladder to accomplish these tasks, it must be able to stretch and accommodate increasing amounts of fluid (urine). This prevents any increases in bladder pressure or rupture of the bladder. This ability of the bladder to stretch is a reflection of the lining of the bladder, called the **urothelium**, and the bladder muscle, the **detrusor**. At a certain point, the bladder muscle must be able to contract strongly and efficiently so that urine can be forced out of the organ and the bladder completely emptied of fluid.

Infants have very little storage because the bladder fills and empties continuously. As an infant matures into a toddler and small child, the lines of communication between the bladder and brain mature, allowing the brain to control the bladder. Thus, when a child is **"potty trained,"** he or she has the ability to hold urine and then voluntarily empty the bladder at a socially acceptable time. During childhood development the bladder grows with the rest of the body. It continues to increase in size until adolescence, when an adult size bladder is achieved. A normal adult bladder capacity is around 10 to 15 ounces (400 cc [cubic centimeters]).

The kidneys produce urine constantly. Urine passes down the **ureter**, which is a long, thin, hollow tubular structure, and drains into the bladder. The wall of the ureter has muscle fibers in it that alternately contract and relax, propelling urine down the ureter into the bladder. This contraction of the ureter along with

Urothelium

type of cell that lines the urinary tract.

Detrusor

the bladder muscle. Coordinated contraction of the detrusor and opening of the bladder outlet allows for normal urination.

Potty training

ability of toddlers to learn how to hold their urine and then voluntarily empty the bladder at a socially acceptable time.

Ureter

a long, thin, hollow tubular structure connecting the kidneys to the bladder so that urine can pass out of the body.

gravity helps ensure that urine moves from the kidney into the bladder. If the bladder pressure is high, the ureter is unable to push urine into the bladder and there is a back-up of urine, called **stasis**, within the ureter and ultimately the kidney. Therefore, while the bladder is storing urine, it also must be "compliant;" that is, it must be able to store urine at a low pressure until the bladder is full. When the bladder is full the muscle contracts, raising the bladder pressure, which leads to the expulsion of urine.

Bladder emptying in the toilet-trained individual is under voluntary control. During bladder filling, the **bladder outlet**, which is the area where the bladder joins the **urethra**, remains closed. This maintains **continence** during bladder filling and storage. During **voiding** there is coordination between the bladder and the urethra such that as the bladder contracts the bladder outlet opens, allowing for the release of urine through the bladder outlet into the urethra. The **urethral sphincter**, a muscle that when contracted closes the urethra, also relaxes during voiding to allow for the passage of urine through the entire urethra. The nervous system controls urination and helps maintain control of urine.

The nervous system is composed of two parts, the central nervous system (brain and spinal cord) and the peripheral nervous system (nerves found in all other parts of the body). Bioelectrical signals are constantly flowing from one nerve to another, telling each cell in the body what to do and when to do it. Some of these signals are consciously done, like when you want to move an arm, and other signals are done without you knowing about them. These unconscious signals drive

The Basics

Stasis
a circumstance in which high pressure in the bladder causes a backup of urine within the ureter and eventually the kidney.

Bladder outlet
area where the bladder joins the urethra.

Urethra
canal leading from the bladder to the body's skin to discharge urine externally.

Continence
ability to retain urine and/or feces until a proper time for their discharge.

Void
to evacuate urine and/or feces.

Urethral sphincter
a muscle that, when contracted, closes the urethra.

most of the complicated bodily functions, for example, blood flow, breathing, etc.

Central nervous system

nerves in the brain and spinal cord; responsible for the starting or preventing urination.

Peripheral nervous system

nerves connecting in the body other than the brain and spinal cord; responsible for the coordination of bladder contraction and urethral relaxation during normal voiding.

Acetylcholine

after the nerve is stimulated, a chemical that is released at the end of one nerve presynaptic cell, and bridges the synapse to stimulate or inhibit the postsynaptic cell.

Muscarinic receptor

a membrane-bound protein that contains a recognition site for acetylcholine.

The **central nervous system** is responsible for starting or preventing urination, whereas the **peripheral nervous system** is responsible for the coordination of bladder contraction and urethral relaxation during normal voiding. The central nervous system is composed of the parasympathetic and sympathetic nervous systems. Activation of the parasympathetic nervous system leads to contraction of the bladder muscle and inhibition of the sympathetic nervous system. The pudendal nerve controls relaxation of the urethral sphincter and the bladder outlet, allowing urine to pass out of the bladder and through the urethra. When the parasympathetic nerves are stimulated, there is a release of a chemical, a neurotransmitter named **acetycholine**, from the end of the nerve. This acetylcholine then attaches to a certain area on the bladder wall, a receptor, and through a series of events stimulates the bladder muscle to contract. Such receptors for acetylcholine are called muscarinic receptors. There are a total of five different **muscarinic receptors** that are located throughout the body. In the bladder, there are two identified muscarinic receptors, M2 and M3. Although the majority of the muscarinic receptors in the bladder are M2 receptors, it appears that the receptor responsible for bladder contractions is the M3 receptor. M2 receptors may have a role in certain abnormal conditions such as spinal cord injury and bladder outlet obstruction. The sympathetic nervous system allows the bladder to hold urine by stimulating the bladder muscle to relax. Storage of urine is also aided by contraction of the bladder neck and the urethral sphincter muscle.

Usually, there is no sensation of bladder fullness until the bladder is about half full. Once the bladder has filled to about half of its capacity, the first sensation of bladder fullness reaches the central nervous system in the brain. At this time, there is an awareness of the need to void, but one can voluntarily suppress this sensation of fullness. An example of this is when you are driving in the car and you feel the urge to urinate, but there are no restrooms around you. Normally, you can suppress this urge and hold onto the urine until you can locate a restroom. At about three quarters capacity there is a stronger desire to urinate.

2. What are normal voiding habits?

It is hard to say what "normal voiding habits" are, since voiding frequency is dependent on fluid intake, the types of fluids that you drink, the medications that you take, and the situations that you are in. Typically, it is thought that the average adult voids roughly every three to four hours while awake and can sleep through the night without having to urinate. Individuals who void more than eight times per day are believed to have **urinary frequency**, and those who get up at night to void have **nocturia**. Remember, however, that if you drink six cups of coffee in the morning, you will need to void frequently due to the diuretic effect of the caffeine. Similarly, if you drink three quarts of fluid per day, you will need to urinate more than eight times in the day. Individuals who take diuretics, sometimes called "water pills," may also experience urinary frequency because of the increased urine volume that the medication produces.

Urinary frequency

having to void eight times or more per day with normal intake of fluids.

Nocturia

having to wake from sleep at night to urinate after a day of normal fluid intake.

3. What problems can occur with bladder function?

The urinary bladder has two main functions: one is to store urine at a low pressure and the other is to expel urine. Problems with bladder function may relate to either of these two functions.

Storage problems include a small capacity bladder, overactive bladder, and poorly compliant bladder. Emptying problems include a poorly contractile bladder, outlet obstruction, and an atonic noncontractile bladder.

Storage Problems

A **small capacity bladder** is one that does not hold much urine. This may be related to fibrosis or scarring within the bladder or from neurologic causes. In this situation, the bladder loses its ability to stretch, so the organ cannot hold the expected amount of urine. With this condition, one tends to void more frequently. Some individuals may have a normal bladder but there appears to be a heightened awareness of bladder filling, leading to urinary frequency.

An **overactive bladder** is one in which the detrusor muscle contracts at times when it should be relaxed, leading to **urinary urgency** (a sudden compelling desire to void that is often difficult to defer), frequency (voiding more than 8 times per day), and possibly nocturia (waking at night one or more times to void). If the contraction is strong enough there may be associated loss of urine, called **urge incontinence**.

A **poorly compliant bladder** is a bladder that holds urine at higher than normal bladder pressures. These

---

Small capacity bladder

a bladder that cannot hold much urine because of fibrosis or scarring or neurological causes.

Overactive bladder

urinary urgency caused by the detrusor muscle contracting at times when it should be relaxed.

Urinary urgency

sudden compelling desire to urinate that often is difficult to defer.

Urge incontinence

unintended leakage or loss of urine into clothing or bedclothes.

Poorly compliant bladder

a bladder that holds urine at higher than normal pressures, causing poor emptying of the kidneys, a back up of urine in the kidneys, and eventually kidney damage.

elevated bladder pressures can cause poor emptying of the kidneys, a backup of urine in the kidneys, and eventually kidney damage.

Emptying Problems

Normal bladder contractility is important in emptying of the bladder. If there is an element of **obstruction/blockage** to the outflow of urine from the bladder (such as with prostate enlargement or strictures, narrowed areas, of the urethra, or medications that affect the urethral musculature), the bladder must be able to generate a higher pressure to overcome the obstruction. In certain cases there may be **poor contractility** of the bladder, where the bladder muscle cannot generate a strong enough squeeze (contraction) and/or sustain the contraction to completely empty the bladder. Poor bladder contractility may result from injury to the nerves supplying the bladder, such as in spinal cord injury, inherited anomalies such as spina bifida (myelomeningocele), chronic overdistention of the bladder, severe long-term outlet obstruction, or medications that affect bladder contractility. Poor contractility of the bladder will lead to increasing amounts of urine left behind in the bladder after voiding. This **"postvoid residual"** urine may lead to urinary tract infections, bladder stones, further distention of the bladder, worsening of the bladder function, and/or elevated bladder pressures that cause dilation of the kidneys and ureter.

An **acontractile bladder** is one that does not contract. This may occur suddenly with no prior history of any troubles with urination, called acute **urinary retention**, or it may be part of a slowly progressive problem. The individual may or may not feel an urge to urinate and

Obstruction

blockage of outflow of urine from the bladder.

Poor contractility

a situation in which the bladder cannot generate and/or sustain the contraction of the organ to completely empty it of urine.

Postvoid residual urine

the amount of urine left behind in the bladder after voiding; if elevated, may lead to urinary tract infection, bladder stones, further distension of the bladder, worsening of bladder functions, and can lead to dilation of the kidneys and ureter.

Acontractile bladder

a bladder that does not contract.

Urinary retention

the inability to urinate on one's own.

will not be able to urinate. It is very important to treat urinary retention immediately to prevent kidney (renal) damage.

4. Is there an age when one is most at risk for urinary incontinence?

Urinary incontinence, which is the inability to prevent the discharge of urine, increases with age for both males and females. Unfortunately, because urinary incontinence is so common in older women, it is sometimes misperceived as a normal and inevitable part of aging. This is not true!

In women, urinary incontinence is present in about 20%–23% who are 30 to 39 years of age. This percentage increases to 25%–30% in those who are 40 to 49 years of age, and this number remains stable until ages 75 to 89, where it increases to 30%–32% and again at 90 years of age, when the prevalence of urinary incontinence is about 35%.

In males, the rate of urinary incontinence increases from 0.7% for males 50 to 59 years of age, to 2.7% for those 60 to 69 years of age, and is 3.4% for those 70 years of age and older. Remember that even though the risk of developing an overactive bladder increases with increasing age, it is not a "normal expected part of aging" and, more importantly, it can be treated.

5. Are there other causes of urinary incontinence besides urge incontinence?

Indeed, there are several other types of urinary incontinence. **Stress urinary incontinence** is the involuntary loss of urine on effort or exertion, such as during

Urinary incontinence

involuntary loss of urine.

Stress urinary incontinence

involuntary loss of urine on effort or exertion, such as during heavy lifting, or on sneezing or coughing.

heavy lifting, or on sneezing or coughing. **Mixed urinary incontinence** is the complaint of involuntary leakage associated with urgency and also with exertion, effort, sneezing, or coughing. **Functional incontinence** is a situation in which the bladder, urethra, and pelvic floor muscles are functioning properly, but physical or mental function interferes with one's ability to independently get to the bathroom on time. Chronic retention may lead to leakage of urine when the bladder is overdistended (expanded beyond its elastic capacity). This usually is the result of obstruction to the outflow of urine due to benign prostate enlargement in men, but may also result from neurologic diseases, poor bladder muscle function, or as a side effect of medications. **Temporary (transient) incontinence** may be caused by illness or medications that increase the volume of urine produced to the point where it interferes with normal urinary tract function.

6. How can I tell the difference between incontinence associated with an overactive bladder (urge incontinence) and stress incontinence?

A review of symptoms and physical examination will allow you and your physician to identify the cause of your urinary leakage. Some women will have both stress and urge incontinence, so there may be more than one cause for urine leakage. An assessment of the presence or absence of the following symptoms will help you to identify the cause of urine leakage (Table 1).

Physical examination of the female includes an examination of your **perineum**. During this part of the examination, you will be asked to strain/bear down

---

Mixed urinary incontinence

involuntary leakage of urine associated with urgency as well as with exertion, effort, sneezing, or coughing.

Functional incontinence

a situation in which the bladder, urethra, and pelvic floor muscles are functioning properly, but physical or mental function interferes with one's ability to independently get to the bathroom on time.

Temporary transient incontinence

leakage of urine caused by illness or medications that increase the volume of urine produced to the point where it interferes with normal urinary tract function that affects normal bladder function..

Perineum

area between the thighs extending from the tail bone (coccyx) to the pubis (between the vulva and anus in the female and scrotum and anus in the male) and lying below the pelvic diaphragm.

The Basics

Table 1   Symptoms found in overactive bladder and stress incontinence

Symptoms	Overactive Bladder	Stress Incontinence
Urgency	Yes	No
Frequency with urgency	Yes	No
Leakage with physical activity (cough, laugh, sneeze)	No	Yes
Amount of urine leaked with each episode	Large, if present	Usually small
Ability to reach toilet in time following an urge to void	No or just barely	Yes
Need to wake up at night to urinate	Often yes	Not often

Radical prostatectomy

a procedure performed for prostate cancer.

Transurethral prostatectomy (TURP)

removal of the prostate through the urethra.

Urodynamic study

a special test used to determine how the bladder and urethral muscles work; includes measuring storage and emptying of the bladder.

(called Valsalva maneuver) and cough while the physician watches for movement of the urethra (hypermobility) and leakage of urine. The presence of hypermobility or leakage with a Valsalva maneuver indicates stress urinary incontinence. Men rarely develop stress incontinence unless they have undergone prior prostate surgery, such as a **radical prostatectomy** for prostate cancer or a **transurethral prostatectomy (TURP)** for benign enlargement of the prostate.

Less commonly, the physician may perform a **urodynamic study** (see Question 58) as an investigative tool to determine the etiology of your urinary symptoms. When an overactive bladder is present, the urodynamic study will often show contractions of the bladder at a time when the bladder muscle should be relaxed (see Figure 1).

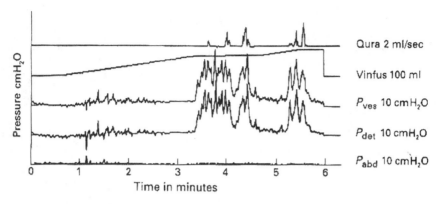

The Basics

Figure 1   Uninhibited contractions in a bladder. (Reprinted with permission from Blandy J, Fowler C: Urology, 2e, 1996. Chapter 24: Bladder Disorders of Junction. Copyright © Blackwell Science, Inc.)

PART TWO

Diagnosis of Overactive Bladder

What is overactive bladder?

What is the natural history of overactive bladder? Is it permanent, can it resolve, or does it come and go?

What causes OAB?

More . . .

7. What is overactive bladder?

Overactive bladder (OAB) is a term that is used to describe a set of symptoms that are suggestive of "uninhibited detrusor contractions." Typically, during bladder filling and storage the bladder muscle remains relaxed to hold urine, and contracts at the time of urination. A contraction of the bladder at a time other than voiding is called an uninhibited bladder contraction. This uninhibited bladder contraction may be felt as a need to urinate or, if the contraction is strong enough or the pelvic floor muscles weakened, there will be loss of urine. If the uninhibited bladder contractions occur frequently, then you will experience urinary frequency.

Overactive bladder (OAB)

urinary urgency caused by the detrusor muscle contracting at times when it should be relaxed.

The symptoms of overactive bladder include: urgency with or without urge incontinence and is often associated with frequency and nocturia:

- Urgency is the complaint of a sudden compelling desire to void, which is often difficult to defer.
- Urge incontinence is the complaint of involuntary loss of urine that is accompanied by or immediately preceded by urgency.
- Urinary frequency is the need to void greater than 8 times in a 24-hour period
- Nocturia is the complaint that the individual has to wake at night one or more times to void.

In a large European epidemiological study, frequency was the most commonly reported symptom in OAB sufferers (85%), followed by urgency (54%), and urge incontinence (36%).

8. Are there medical conditions that may cause or mimic overactive bladder?

There are a variety of conditions that may produce symptoms typical of overactive bladder. Transient or reversible conditions include urinary tract infection, estrogen deficiency in the female, drug side effects (Table 2), excessive urine output, restricted mobility, severe constipation, and altered mental status (Table 3). Other conditions that can contribute to, or may be associated with overactive bladder include: obstruction to the outflow of urine from the bladder, pelvic prolapse (descent of the bladder and other pelvic organs out of the pelvis), and significant stress incontinence.

Acute (i.e., sudden onset of symptoms) and potentially treatable causes of urinary incontinence include (acronym: DIAPPERS):

- **D**elirium—confusion
- **I**nfection
- **A**trophic vaginitis—low or absent estrogen levels before or after menopause, after hysterectomy and oophorectomy
- **P**harmaceutical agents—medications
- **P**sychologic—depression, dementia
- **E**xcess urine output—secondary to increased fluid intake, increased renal production of urine, or overflow incontinence
- **R**estricted mobility—difficulty with ambulation (walking) related to musculoskeletal problems or environmental factors
- **S**tool impaction—significant constipation

Atrophic vaginitis

low or absent estrogen levels before or after menopause, after hysterectomy and oophorectomy.

15

Table 2   Medications that may cause side effects that contribute to urinary incontinence

Drug Class	Side Effects
Alcohol	Polyuria, frequency, urgency, sedation, delirium
Alpha-agonists (e.g., pseudoephedrine, ephedrine)	Urinary retention
Alpha-blockers (e.g., tamsulosin (Flomax), doxazosin (Cardura), terazosin (Hytrin))	Urethral relaxation
ACE inhibitors, type I	Diuresis, cough with relaxation of pelvic floor
Anticholinergics (e.g., Oxybutynin, Detrol, Ditropan)	Urinary retention, overflow incontinence, stool impaction
Antidepressants (e.g., imipramine [Tofranil])	See anticholinergic side effects, sedation
Antiparkinsonism medications	Urinary urgency, constipation
Antipsychotics	See anticholinergic side effects, sedation, rigidity
Beta-agonists	Urinary retention
Caffeine	Bladder irritability that may aggravate or cause urge incontinence
Calcium-channel blockers	Urinary retention
Diuretics	Polyuria, urinary frequency, urgency
Sedatives/hypnotics	Sedation, delirium, immobility

Table 3   Management of conditions that cause reversible urinary incontinence

Condition	Management
Difficulty getting to or unwillingness to go to the toilet	
Delirium	Identification and management of the cause of the confused state of mind
Impaired mobility	Regular toileting, use of toilet substitutes (i.e., bedside commode, urinal)
Psychological problems	Appropriate psychological therapy
Drug side effects	If appropriate, discontinuation or decreased dosage of the drug, or changing to an alternative drug
Increased urine production	
Hyperglycemia	Improved control of blood sugars
Hypercalcemia	Treatment of the cause of the hypercalcemia
Excess fluid intake	Restriction of fluid intake and avoidance of caffeinated fluids
Fluid overload	
Venous insufficiency with Lower extremity edema	Support hose (TEDs), elevation of legs, low sodium diet
Congestive heart failure	Medical therapy to optimize cardiac function
Urinary tract infection	Antibiotic therapy
Atrophic vaginitis/ urethritis	Topical estrogen therapy if not at risk for use of estrogen therapy
Stool impaction	Disimpaction (manual removal of stool), institution of therapy to prevent constipation including: increased fiber and fluids, stool softeners, and/or laxatives if needed

9. What causes overactive bladder?

The primary cause of overactive bladder is not well defined. The mechanism for overactivity of the bladder may be related to a problem with nerves, a neurogenic cause (i.e., something starting from or caused by the nerves themselves), a problem with the bladder muscle itself, or a myogenic cause, but there also may be other causes. The central nervous system, which encompasses the brain and the spinal cord, controls bladder function in a manner similar to an on-off circuit that you are able to voluntarily control. Damage to certain areas of the brain and spinal cord may alter this on-off circuit and lead to bladder overactivity. Neurological conditions that may be associated with overactive bladder include Parkinson's disease, multiple sclerosis, and spinal cord injury. Conditions that may lead to alterations in the bladder muscle function include bladder outlet obstruction, such as in men with benign enlargement of the prostate gland (BPH), or aging. Specialized studies of bladder function, called urodynamic studies (discussed in Question 58), have demonstrated an age-related decrease in the size of the bladder, and an increased incidence of uninhibited bladder contractions, a decreased force of the urine stream, and a decreased volume of urine voided along with incomplete bladder emptying. Changes in the muscarinic receptors in the bladder may also occur with aging. In a European study, some aspects of diet and lifestyle were associated with an increased risk of developing overactive bladder. These factors included soda intake, being overweight or obese, and smoking.

Lastly, changes in the **afferent pathway** may cause the bladder to be overactive. Nerves within the bladder wall and lining (urothelium) respond to stretching of the bladder (such as during bladder filling and noxious

Afferent pathway

messages (nerve impulse signals) inflowing to the central nervous system (brain and spinal cord).

stimuli) by sending messages (nerve impulses) to the brain via the spinal cord, and these messages tell the brain that the bladder needs to respond. The brain then sends impulses to the bladder (**efferent pathway**) to tell the bladder to contract. Thus, abnormalities in the afferent pathway may lead to overactivity in the efferent pathway, which is responsible for bladder contractions.

Efferent pathway

messages (nerve impulse signals) out-flowing from the central nervous system to the peripheral nervous system.

10. How common is overactive bladder?

Overactive bladder is a very common condition. Previous studies estimated that approximately 16% of Americans suffered from overactive bladder and that worldwide between 50 and 100 million individuals suffered from overactive bladder. More recent studies suggest that the prevalence of overactive bladder may be even greater. Overactive bladder affects both males and females. The prevalence of overactive bladder increases with age for both males and females (Figure 2). Overactive bladder

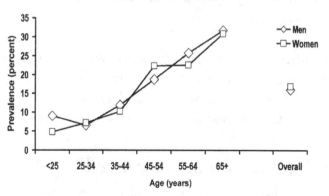

Prevalence of OAB by Age

Data from the National Overactive BLadder Evaluation (NOBLE) Research Program

Figure 2   Relationship between overactive bladder and age. (Adapted from Stewart WF, van Rooten JB, Cundiff GW, Abrams P, Hezzog AR et al. Prevalence of Overactive Bladder in US. World J Urol 2002. Reprinted with permission from Springer-Verlag).

tends to develop in men over the age of 60 years, whereas in women it tends to develop in the mid 40s, although it may develop at any time in both sexes. Urge incontinence is more frequently seen in women (9.3% females with OAB) than males (2.6% males with OAB). Thus, women have a greater chance of being "OAB wet" and men are more likely to be "OAB dry."

11. What is the natural history of overactive bladder? Is it permanent, can it resolve, or does it come and go?

There is little information regarding the natural history of overactive bladder. The few studies that are available suggest that overactive bladder is a chronic condition in adults that persists symptomatically. In one study that followed patients with overactive bladder for as long as 10 years, bladder overactivity persisted in 69% of the individuals, regardless of their treatment. There may be exacerbations and improvements in your symptoms depending on lifestyle and dietary changes.

In children it appears that overactive bladder is a transient condition that resolves with time. There are no long-term studies, however, to determine whether these children develop symptoms again later in life.

12. Is overactive bladder hereditary?

There is little information available regarding the genetics of overactive bladder. In studies of twins, there was a suggestion that OAB with urge incontinence may be hereditary. In children with OAB there is often a family member with OAB. In a recent study of female urinary incontinence, hereditary factors did appear to play a role in the development of urinary incontinence in women. The study found that there was an increased risk for any type of incontinence, that is, stress or mixed (stress plus urge), and severe symptoms for women whose mothers or older sisters were incontinent.

13. What is the impact of overactive bladder?

Overactive bladder has a negative effect on quality of life. It is associated with additional medical comorbidities (i.e., abnormal, pathologic, or diseased) and has a huge economic impact.

Studies evaluating the effect of overactive bladder and urge incontinence on quality of life have demonstrated that urge incontinence has a greater negative effect on quality of life than stress incontinence. This is understandable when one considers that with stress incontinence the individual has an element of control. If he or she avoids coughing, laughing, sneezing, or exertion, then leaking can be avoided. With urge, however, there is no warning or control.

When compared to several other disease states, individuals with urge incontinence believed that they had a worse quality of life in several quality-of-life parameters than individuals who had diabetes mellitus. Only depressed patients rated their quality of life worse than individuals with urge incontinence.

Overactive bladder and urinary incontinence may affect one's quality of life in a variety of ways:

- Psychological—may lead to guilt/depression, loss of self-esteem and fear of being a burden, and fear of lack of bladder control or the smell of urine odor.
- Social—may lead to a reduction in social interactions, and limit travel to planning around toilet accessibility.
- Domestic—there is a need for specialized pads and protective underwear; if the individual is elderly, he or she may have to depend on a caregiver to obtain these items.
- Occupational—may lead to absences from work, decreased productivity, and difficulties with colleagues at work.
- Sexual—may lead to avoidance of sexual activity and intimacy.
- Physical—may lead to limitation or cessation of physical activity, particularly in those individuals who suffer from mixed incontinence.

Studies have demonstrated that urinary incontinence is the reason for nursing home admission in about 50% of nursing home patients. In the elderly, urinary incontinence is associated with an increased risk of urinary tract infections, skin infections, and irritation. Furthermore, there is an association between overactive bladder and urinary incontinence with risk of falls and bone fractures in older women. The risk of falls was 26% and fractures 34% in the elderly with overactive bladder.

The overall economic burden of urge incontinence is extremely high. In 1995, it was estimated to be 17.5 billion dollars, which exceeded the economic burden for breast cancer or pneumonia. This economic burden reflects the costs of pads and diapers, laundry costs, treatment for urinary tract infections and skin infections/irritation, and medical therapy for overactive bladder. In addition, there are additional costs that are difficult to measure, such as the time spent by a caregiver and nursing home care related to urinary incontinence.

14. Is overactive bladder treatable?

Yes, overactive bladder is treatable. Most individuals will note a significant improvement in their symptoms with a combination of behavioral modification and medical therapy (see Questions 25–34). Although each of these therapies is effective alone, the best results are noted when they are used in combination. Those individuals who do not improve with medical therapy and behavioral modification, or for whom medical therapy is contraindicated (i.e., medically inappropriate) may be treated with other forms of therapy, including sacral neuromodulation and intravesical capsaicin and intravesical resiniferatoxin (see Questions 35–38). Rarely, the overactive bladder symptoms may be refractory to these therapies (i.e., the therapy doesn't work). Then an injection of botulinum toxin into the bladder, bladder augmentation procedures, or **bladder denervation** procedures may be considered (see Questions 39–48).

When you discuss therapy for overactive bladder, it is important that you and your physician discuss the expectations of the treatment. For example, if you are currently voiding 20 times per day and have 5 incontinent episodes per day, a reasonable expectation may be a reduction in your urinary frequency and incontinence

Bladder denervation

techniques to deaden or eliminate the nerves in the urethra, bladder, or rectum in an effort to interrupt the nerve supply to the bladder and stop bladder contractions.

episodes by 50%. If you are expecting to be dry all the time and void 6 times per day with therapy, this may not be realistic with medical therapy.

15. Is overactive bladder curable?

Medical therapy in combination with behavioral modification improves overactive bladder symptoms in up to 85% of individuals. This does not mean that all of these individuals are dry and that none of them continue to experience urgency and frequency. Medical therapy "cures" individuals in fewer than 25% of cases. In addition, it is important to remember that medical therapy does not cause any permanent or long-standing changes. So if you are doing well on medical therapy and suddenly stop the therapy, the likelihood is that your overactive bladder symptoms will return. There are no long-term studies available on neuromodulation to assess whether or not it "cures" an overactive bladder. Neither intravesical capsaicin/resiniferatoxin nor injection of botulinum toxin provide for permanent cure, and each will need to be repeated periodically. Permanent denervation procedures and bladder augmentation may permanently "cure" overactive bladder.

16. Can men have prostate problems and overactive bladder or is it all just related to the prostate?

Lower urinary tract symptoms (LUTS) is a term used to describe two types of lower urinary tract symptoms: obstructive and irritative symptoms. Men with enlarged prostates will often present with voiding symptoms such as a slow stream, hesitancy, intermittent stream, and straining; they may also experience

Lower urinary tract symptoms (LUTS)
term used to describe destructive and irritative voiding symptoms.

postvoiding dribbling. These symptoms are often related to the obstruction to the outflow of urine from the enlarged prostate. Approximately 40% to 60% of men with prostatic enlargement and bladder outlet obstruction have irritative symptoms including daytime frequency, nocturia, urgency, and less commonly urge incontinence. These irritative symptoms are suggestive of an overactive bladder. The fact that up to 38% of men with benign enlargement of the prostate who undergo surgical treatment for their prostatic enlargement still suffer from irritative symptoms after the treatment suggests that truly they have two conditions: obstruction due to the prostatic enlargement and overactive bladder. In some individuals, however, treatment of the prostatic enlargement will improve the overactive bladder symptoms. Why this occurs is not fully understood.

Because it appears that men with prostatic enlargement can suffer from symptoms related to the obstruction and may also have overactive bladder, current studies are underway that are looking at the use of medical therapy to treat both of these symptoms. Limited studies have demonstrated that it is feasible to use a combination of medications used for prostatic enlargement, such as alpha blockers (examples include doxazosin [Cardura], terazosin [Hytrin] and tamsulosin) and anticholinergics (tolterodine, oxybutynin).

17. Is waking up at night caused by overactive bladder?

Nocturia is defined as the complaint that an individual has to wake at night one or more times to void. Nocturia is very common, and it appears that the incidence and severity increases as one gets older. In one European study, 10% of the general population age 20 years and older suffered from nocturia two or more times per night. In addition, this study demonstrated that nocturia has a significant impact on one's quality of life, and that there was a correlation between the number of times one awakened at night to void and the impact on quality of life. Nocturia is often present with overactive bladder, but there are several other important causes including:

- Cardiovascular disease, including congestive heart failure and circulatory problems
- Diabetes mellitus
- Diabetes insipidus, which is a condition that is either related to a brain or kidney problem and results in the overproduction of urine
- Sleep apnea, which is a breathing problem that occurs during sleep
- Lower urinary tract obstruction such as that related to prostate enlargement
- Primary sleep disorders
- Behavioral and environmental factors
- Nocturnal polyuria, whereby the urine output over the course of the entire day is normal, but the urine output at night is in excess of what is normal
- Polyuria, whereby the total urine output for the entire day is excessive

Frequency volume chart

a document plotting the amount of urine, and number of times an individual urinates over a period of time.

To determine whether the nocturia is related to overactive bladder requires that your physician review your history, medications, and a **frequency volume chart**. A frequency volume chart or bladder diary allows your physician to determine the potential cause of your nocturia (see Question 27). Treatment of the nocturia will vary with the cause. Preliminary studies have demonstrated, however, that if the cause of the nocturia is overactive bladder, the use of anticholinergics will help to decrease the number of times that you will need to void at night.

18. How is overactive bladder diagnosed?

Overactive bladder (OAB) is a condition with symptoms that are suggestive of uninhibited bladder contractions, in the setting of no identifiable metabolic or pathologic conditions that mimic or cause overactive bladder. The evaluation has two purposes: (1) to determine whether the individual's symptoms are suggestive of OAB, and (2) to rule out those metabolic or pathologic conditions that may cause or mimic OAB. The initial evaluation starts with an analysis of your symptoms to determine whether they are consistent with OAB. Remember, those individuals with OAB suffer from urgency with or without urge incontinence and will often have frequency and nocturia (see Question 6). Simplified bladder health questionnaires allow the physician to screen for possible bladder troubles. The following questions are often asked.

Over the past four weeks:

- Did you wake up at night to urinate two or more times?
- Did you have a sudden and uncomfortable feeling that you had to urinate soon?
- Were you bothered or concerned about bladder control?
- Did you lose or leak urine for any reason?
- Did you wear a pad or other material to absorb urine that you may have lost?

Symptom Assessment

A symptom assessment will focus on your urinary symptoms, and ask how often you urinate, do you have urgency, and if there is leakage. The physician will ask whether straining, coughing, laughing, or sneezing induces leakage. It is often helpful for you to complete a voiding diary over several days to better clarify your urinary symptoms (see Question 27). In addition, your doctor will want to know how bothered you are by these symptoms. If you are not bothered, then unless you are suffering from recurrent urinary tract or skin infections there is no need to treat you. During the symptom assessment, the doctor will try to determine whether your symptoms are suggestive of OAB, stress incontinence, or a combination of two, which is mixed urinary incontinence. As part of your symptom assessment, your doctor may ask you to complete a voiding diary for three to five days to better understand your fluid intake and symptoms (Figure 3).

History and Physical Examination

A medical history and physical examination and a urinalysis are helpful in ruling out other conditions that mimic or cause OAB (see Question 7). During the history component, your doctor will want to know about your prior and current medical and surgical histories, what medications you are taking, and if you have allergies. Questions about the medical status of your relatives may be asked. In addition, several questions pertaining to dietary and lifestyle issues will be asked. These may include: how much fluids you typically drink during the day, how much caffeinated fluids you drink, your occupation, and your ease of access to restrooms at work. The physical examination will focus

Optional Tools for Consideration: Voiding Log/Bladder Diary

Day 1   Date: __/__/__   Number of pads used today:____

TIME	FLUIDS		URINATION					ACCIDENTS		
	What did you drink?	How much?	How many times?	How much each time? (S=small, M=moderate, L=large)	Did you have to rush to the bathroom?	Did you hurt yourself or fall down rushing to the bathroom?	What activity did it Interrupt?	Did you have any accidents this time? (Sudden loss of urine)	How much urine did you leak? (S=small, M=moderate, L=large)	What were you doing at the time? (Exercising, sleeping, relaxing, etc.)
SAMPLE 12 PM	Juice	Tall glass	1	(S) M L	(Yes) No	Yes (No)	Walking the dog	(Yes) No	(S) M L	Gardening
				S M L	Yes No	Yes No		Yes No	S M L	
				S M L	Yes No	Yes No		Yes No	S M L	
				S M L	Yes No	Yes No		Yes No	S M L	
				S M L	Yes No	Yes No		Yes No	S M L	
				S M L	Yes No	Yes No		Yes No	S M L	
				S M L	Yes No	Yes No		Yes No	S M L	
				S M L	Yes No	Yes No		Yes No	S M L	
				S M L	Yes No	Yes No		Yes No	S M L	
				S M L	Yes No	Yes No		Yes No	S M L	

Notes:_____   13

Figure 3   Sample of a voiding diary.

on your lower abdomen and perineum. Often a brief neurological evaluation will be included. The doctor will palpate your lower abdomen to see if your bladder is distended. In women, a pelvic examination is performed to determine if there is significant **pelvic prolapse**. During the examination of the perineum in women, the physician may ask you to strain/bear down or cough to determine if there is any loss of control of urine. Some physicians may put a small Q-tip into the urethra and then ask you to strain to see if there is a significant deflection of the Q-tip suggestive of stress urinary incontinence. A rectal examination is often performed to check anal muscle tone. In males, the rectal examination includes a prostate examination to check the size of the prostate, and to determine if

Pelvic prolapse
a weakening in the web of muscles at the base of the pelvis.

29

there are nodules that may indicate the presence of prostate cancer.

Urinalysis

A **urinalysis** is a helpful test to rule out a urinary tract infection. In addition, the presence of red blood cells in the urine in the absence of a urinary tract infection would require further evaluation. The presence of a bladder tumor or stone as the cause of the blood cells in the urine and the voiding symptoms needs to ruled out. The presence of an excessive amount of glucose in the urine would prompt further evaluation for diabetes, and the presence of an excessive amount of protein in the urine would prompt further evaluation for kidney diseases. A very dilute urine is suggestive of either drinking excessive amounts of fluid or an inability of the kidney to hold fluids back.

Additional Studies

Depending on your age, voiding symptoms, and prior medical and surgical history, you may need additional studies. In men with symptoms suggestive of obstruction from an enlarged prostate, elderly patients, patients with recurrent urinary tract infections, and those with neurological diseases, the doctor may perform a bladder scan after the individual has urinated to ensure that the bladder is emptying properly. Less commonly, a catheter may be passed through the urethra into the bladder to drain the bladder and measure the postvoid urine volume. The bladder scan postvoid residual determination is performed by having the individual urinate and then placing a small ultrasound probe on the lower abdomen to determine if there is any fluid (urine) remaining in the bladder. The machine will calculate an estimated volume of urine in the bladder. Younger individuals should be able to empty their bladder to completion. As one gets older, there is an anticipated small amount of urine that may be left behind after urinating. Postvoid residuals greater than 150 cc are considered to be abnormal and suggestive of either outlet obstruction or poor bladder function. Rarely will any additional studies be needed. Those individuals with red blood cells in the urine will need to undergo a cystoscopy. Cystoscopy is the procedure in which the bladder and urethra are examined through a narrow telescope-like device that is passed through the urethra into the bladder. In those individuals with complex medical problems, prior bladder or urethral surgery, and those who have failed prior therapies for overactive bladder, a urodynamic study may be indicated (see Question 58).

PART THREE

Treatment of Overactive Bladder

What are the options for treating overactive bladder?

What are pelvic floor muscle exercises
(Kegel exercises)?

What is neuromodulation/sacral nerve stimulation?

What is bladder augmentation?

More . . .

19. What are the treatment options for overactive bladder?

There are a variety of treatment options available for the management of overactive bladder. These options vary from less invasive therapies, such as behavioral therapy and oral therapies, to more invasive therapies, such as intravesical therapies and surgical treatments. Typically you begin with the less invasive therapies first, reserving the surgical and intravesical therapies for those who fail behavioral and oral therapies.

First-line therapies for the management of overactive bladder include:

* Behavioral therapy (Figure 4)
* Pharmacologic therapy—medications

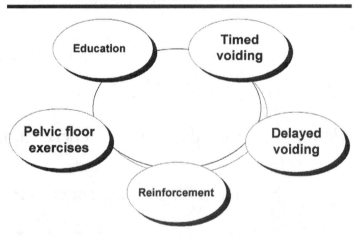

Figure 4   Types of behavioral therapy and management of symptoms.

Second-line therapies include:

- Intravesical therapy—capsaicin and resiniferatoxin
- Sacral neuromodulation—electrical stimulation
- Injection of botulinum toxin into the bladder

Third-line therapies include:

- Bladder augmentation
- Urinary diversion
- Bladder denervation procedures

This section discusses the above options individually in detail.

NONOPERATIVE OPTIONS

20. What medications are available to treat overactive bladder?

There are a variety of medications that are currently approved by the Food and Drug Administration (FDA). The goal of all of these medications is the suppression of the uninhibited bladder contractions, which will lead to less urinary frequency, urgency, and urge incontinence episodes. Currently, antimuscarinic agents are the gold standard for the pharmacologic management of overactive bladder. Historically, **antimuscarinics** have been demonstrated to be effective in increasing bladder capacity and inhibiting uninhibited bladder contractions; however, their use has been limited due to a high incidence of side effects. Since OAB is a condition that adversely affects quality of life, it is important to have a medical therapy that improves the

Antimuscarinic agents

a type of medication that produces effects that stimulate the parasympathetic receptor, which is involved in the control of bladder muscle contraction.

symptoms of OAB, but does not cause side effects that will have a significant negative effect on quality of life. Thus, the major emphasis on the development of new medical therapies is on decreasing the side effect profile of the medications while maintaining the efficacy of the medication. A variety of novel ways of administering drugs have been utilized to help in this endeavor. Drugs may be given in several different ways: in multiple doses per day in the traditional delivery system, the pill or capsule; in a sustained release/long-acting formulation that allows for once a day dosing; a **transdermal** (skin patch) system; or as an **intravesical** (placed directly into the bladder) preparation.

Transdermal
medication is delivered to the body by a skin patch.

Intravesical
medication placed directly into the bladder.

21. How do antimuscarinics work to decrease overactive bladder symptoms?

There are currently five different muscarinic receptors in the body and the bladder contains two of them: M2 and M3.

The M3 receptors are responsible for detrusor contraction, yet they comprise only a small percentage of the muscarinic receptors in the bladder (20%). When the parasympathetic nerves release acetylcholine, the chemical binds to the M3 receptor and, through a complex interaction involving calcium, the bladder muscle is stimulated to contract.

The M2 receptor is the most abundant receptor in the bladder (80%), but it appears to only have a role in bladder muscle activity in certain pathologic states such as spinal cord injury and outlet obstruction. The actual role of the M2 receptor in human bladders is not fully understood. When stimulated, the M2 receptor indirectly facilitates bladder contraction by blocking relaxation of the bladder muscle. Muscarinic receptors also are located on the nerve endings, and these may have a role in bladder contractility, too.

There are M1 receptors on the nerve endings that when activated stimulate the release of acetylcholine and M2/M4 receptors, which may inhibit the release of acetycholine depending on the degree of stimulation.

22. Is there anyone who should not take an antimuscarinic (anticholinergic) medication?

Antimuscarinic therapy should not be used in individuals with urinary retention, poor stomach emptying, those with narrow angle glaucoma, or anyone at risk of developing any one of these conditions. If you have glaucoma, the safest thing to do is to check with your eye doctor prior to starting an antimuscarinic. Care should be taken in using antimuscarinics in individuals with liver or kidney failure. Question 24 discusses the side effects of this therapy.

23. What are the available antimuscarinics/anticholinergics?

Currently used medications in the United States for the treatment of overactive bladder include: oxybutynin, Ditropan XL, transdermal oxybutynin (Oxytrol), tolterodine (Detrol), Detrol LA, propantheline, hyoscyamine, flavoxate, and imipramine. Recently approved medications include trospium chloride (Sanctura, Indevus), solifenacin (Vesicare, Yamanouchi), and darifenacin (Enablex, Novartis). All of these medications share a similar efficacy (benefits and effectiveness). The medications differ in their muscarinic receptor selectivity, organ selectivity, dosing regimen, metabolism, and side effect profile. The selection of the most appropriate drug for each individual thus will need to take into account these differences and how they will affect each individual patient.

Oxybutynin

Oxybutynin is one of the oldest medical therapies for overactive bladder. Oxybutynin is a chemical that is noted to have several different effects: it has been shown to be an antimuscarinic, to have direct effects on the bladder smooth muscle, and also to have anesthetic properties. In the usual dosing regimens it appears that its effects are the result of its antimuscarinic properties. However, very large doses, more than those that are routinely used, are required to achieve a direct muscle relaxant effect, and the anesthetic effect is probably only helpful in those individuals who place the oxybutynin directly into their bladder via a catheter. Oxybutynin has more of an affinity for the M1 and M3 receptors than the M2, M4, and M5 receptors. In humans, oxybutynin has a higher affinity for the salivary gland than the bladder muscarinic receptors.

Oxybutynin may be administered in several ways. Generic oxybutynin is often given on a three times a day basis, but may be given as infrequently as once a day and as frequently as four times a day. Typically, individuals start with a 5 mg tablet on a twice a day or three times a day regimen. Generic oxybutynin has been shown to be an effective medication in the treatment of OAB. It has been shown to decrease urinary frequency, urinary urgency, and urge incontinence episodes. Unfortunately, a large amount of the oxybutynin is metabolized by the liver, leading to a high level of the metabolite. The metabolite of oxybutynin causes more dry mouth than oxybutynin itself, which has led to a problem historically with compliance.

Ditropan XL

The long-acting formulation of oxybutynin, ditropan XL, is taken only once per day. There are several different strengths (5 mg, 10 mg, and 15 mg capsules), and it may be titrated up to 30 mg per day as needed. Essentially the dose of ditropan XL is the same as the total daily dose of oxybutynin. For example, if an individual was taking oxybutynin at 5 mg three times a day, then he/she would take one ditropan XL 15-mg capsule per day. The advantages of the once-daily dose include ease of use and a lower incidence of side effects (see Question 24). The different capsule strengths allow for flexibility and dose titration. The capsule of ditropan XL is unique in that there is a small laser-drilled hole in the capsule. As fluid is absorbed into the capsule, the drug is pushed out of the hole. The capsule itself does not break down, so don't be alarmed if you see it floating in the toilet bowl or in your colostomy bag if you have a bowel bag. This capsule should not be crushed or cut as it will no longer function as a long-acting medication.

Transdermal Oxybutynin

A new form of delivery of oxybutynin is transdermal oxybutynin, the skin patch. The oxybutynin is contained within a thin, almost clear adhesive patch that is attached to the skin on a twice-weekly basis. The patch may be applied to the abdomen, buttock, or the hip. A new application site should be used with each new patch to avoid re-application to the same area within a seven-day period. There is no difference in the absorption of the oxybutynin when the patch is applied to different areas of the body. Each patch contains a total of 36 mg of oxybutynin and releases about 3.9 mg of oxybutynin per day through the skin. After application of the first patch, it takes 24 (one day) to 48 hours (two days) to reach the systemic level of 3 to 4 mg, and the concentration remains steady for approximately 96 hours. Thus, the patch cannot be used on an as-needed basis (called "prn"). Similar to the once-daily preparation, the patch decreases the amount of oxybutynin that is metabolized by the liver and thus decreases the amount of the active metabolite. This reduction in the amount of the active metabolite can improve the tolerability by decreasing the incidence and severity of dry mouth.

Advantages of transdermal oxybutynin include its ease of use and decreased anticholinergic side effect profile compared to oxybutynin. In 99.3% of individuals, the patch completely adheres well to the skin. In some individuals, skin irritation at the patch application site may occur; 8% develop redness at the site of patch application and 17% develop itchiness at the site. Skin irritation may be a more significant problem in the elderly, who have thin, sensitive skin.

Tolterodine (Detrol)

Tolterodine is the first antimuscarinic medication that was developed solely for its use in overactive bladder. Most of the medications currently used for overactive bladder were actually first developed for use for irritable bowel syndrome. Tolterodine, on the other hand, was first used in the treatment of overactive bladder. Unlike oxybutynin, tolterodine is not selective for a particular muscarinic receptor and, thus, it affects M1, M2, and M3 receptors. It is unique in that it is organ selective; this means that it has a higher affinity or "stickiness" for the muscarinic receptors in the bladder compared to other organ systems, particularly the salivary gland. This selectivity for the bladder over the salivary gland is associated with a much lower incidence of dry mouth. In addition, there is a lower incidence of constipation with tolterodine compared to oxybutynin (see Table 4). Unlike oxybutynin, the active metabolite of tolterodine shares the same properties as the parent compound. The chemical structure of tolterodine makes it less able to penetrate the brain compared to oxybutynin. When brain wave function is measured by a machine known as an electroencephalograph (which produces electroencephalograms, EEGs), tolterodine is associated with fewer changes than oxybutynin. The clinical significance of these EEG changes is not well described. Tolterodine is available in two formulations, a twice-a-day formulation and a once-a-day formulation (Detrol LA). The usual daily dose is 2-mg orally twice a day or one 4-mg Detrol LA capsule. Lower doses, 1 mg orally twice-a-day or one 2 mg Detrol LA capsule, are used in the elderly.

Detrol LA

Unlike Ditropan XL, the capsule itself of tolterodine is not responsible for is extended release action. Rather, inside the Detrol LA capsule, there are very tiny balls (microspheres) containing the medication that provide for its sustained release action. The advantages of the once-a-day preparation include ease of use, improved compliance, and a stabilization of the peak (the highest

Table 4 More commonly used anticholinergics for overactive bladder

Drug	Dosage	Side Effect		
		Dry Mouth	Constipation	CNS
Oxybutynin	2.5–5 mg t.i.d.	++++	++++	Crosses BBB
Oxybutynin XL	5–30 mg q.d.	++–+++	++–+++	Crosses BBB
Transdermal oxybutynin	36 mg patch 2 ×/week	+	+	Crosses BBB
Tolterodine	1–2 mg b.i.d.	++	++	Less likely to cross BBB
Tolterodine LA	2–4 mg q.d.	++	++	Less likely to cross BBB
Trospium chloride	20 mg PO b.i.d.	++	++	Doesn't cross BBB
Darifenacin	7.5–15 mg q.d.	++–+++	++	No effect on brain
Solifenacin	5–10 mg q.d.	++	+++	Unknown

Abbreviations are: t.i.d., three times per day; BBB, blood brain barrier (agents that cross the blood brain barrier are able to enter the brain, and if they interact with certain muscarinic receptors, they may cause central nervous system effects such as cognitive dysfunction, that is, memory problems); q.d., every day; b.i.d., twice a day; PO, by mouth (per os); FDA, Federal Drug Administration.

amount of drug in the bloodstream) and trough (the lowest amount of drug in the bloodstream prior to taking the next dose) levels of the drug in the patient's bloodstream. The decrease in the peak level may account for its better side effect profile when compared to the twice-a-day formulation. The increase in the trough may account for a slightly better result (**efficacy**) for the extended release preparation. Detrol LA has been shown to improve urgency, allowing an increasing number of individuals to finish tasks and remain dry before rushing to the bathroom when the symptom of urgency occurs.

Efficacy
extent to which a specific intervention, procedure, regimen, or service produces a beneficial result under ideal conditions.

Trospium Chloride

Trospium chloride (Sanctura, Indevus) is an antimuscarinic that is currently being used in Europe for overactive bladder and recently was approved for use in the United States by the FDA. Trospium chloride's chemical structure is such that it is unlikely to penetrate the brain and thus does not appear to affect cognitive function. Trospium chloride is usually administered as 20 mg orally twice a day. Trospium chloride should not be taken within one hour of eating. An advantage of this medication is that it has little reaction with other medications. If the trospium chloride is going to be effective, you can expect to see a response as soon as one week after starting the therapy. The most frequently reported side effects of trospium chloride are dry mouth (21.8%–54%) and constipation (9.5%). The efficacy of trospium chloride is similar to that of oxybutynin and tolterodine.

Solifenacin

Solifenacin (Vesicare, Yamanouchi) is another antimuscarinic that has been recently approved by the FDA for use in overactive bladder. It appears to have a tissue preference for the bladder over the salivary gland. It is a once-daily oral medication and is available in two doses, 5 mg and 10 mg. It is a medication that was originally developed for use in irritable bowel syndrome and later demonstrated to be effective for overactive bladder. Unlike many of the other anticholinergics, it has a long half-life and it takes about one week after starting the drug regimen to develop an adequate drug level to be effective. Solifenacin shows a similar efficacy to oxybutynin and tolterodine. As with other antimuscarinics, the most common side effect of solifenacin is dry mouth, as 14% who are taking 5 mg and 21.3% with 10 mg doses also have dry mouth. Whether solifenacin is able to penetrate the brain is unknown at present. The tablet cannot be crushed or cut.

Darifenacin

Darifenacin (Enablex, Novartis) is an antimuscarinic agent that is selective for the M3 receptor. This muscarinic receptor is the receptor responsible for bladder contractility in the normal bladder. Darfenacin is available in two, once a day doses, 7.5 mg and 15 mg, which will allow for dose titration and dose flexability. Darifenacin has been shown to increase the warning time compared to placebo. **Warning time** is defined as the duration between the individual's initial perception of urinary urgency and the onset of voiding. A longer warning time allows the individual to have more bladder control. Since darifenacin is an M3 receptor-selective agent, theoretically it should not have an effect on the brain. This has been demonstrated in cognitive function and memory testing studies. In an animal model, darifenacin was shown to have more affinity for the bladder than the salivary gland and, thus, it appears to be a bladder selective medication. This is supported clinically by a rela-

Warning time
duration of time between the individual's initial perception of urinary urgency and the onset of voiding.

tively lower incidence of dry mouth in the human studies, because 30% who took the 7.5 mg dose and 39% with the 15 mg dose experienced dry mouth. The incidence of constipation is similar to that of other anticholinergic medications: 12% with the 7.5 mg and 15% with the 15 mg dose. Its M3 receptor selectivity also prevents it from having an effect on the heart rate. The efficacy of darifenacin is similar to that of the other approved anticholinergics/antimuscarinics. The tablet cannot be crushed or cut.

Less commonly used medications

Propantheline bromide. Probanthine is a nonselective antimuscarinic that is usually given in doses of 15 to 30 mg orally four times a day. Each individual may require a different dose, so it is recommend that you titrate to the dose that produces the desired results with tolerable side effects. Some individuals will require even higher doses to achieve an acceptable response. Individual responses vary, and a review of five randomized controlled studies demonstrated that the use of probanthine decreased urgency by 0% to 53%.

Antidepressants

Several antidepressants have been shown to be effective in the treatment of overactive bladder. **Imipramine** is the antidepressant that is the most commonly used for overactive bladder. It is not clear how imipramine actually affects overactive bladder. It does possess antimuscarinic properties and it prevents the reuptake of two neurotransmitters in the brain: serotonin and noradrenaline. Both serotonin and noradrenaline are involved in the complex interactions related to normal bladder filling and emptying. Dosing of imipramine varies. Imipramine can have

Imipramine

an antidepressant medication used for overactive bladder; it has antimuscarinic properties and acts on two neurotransmitters in the brain (sertotonin and noradrenaline) involved in the complex interactions related to normal bladder filling and emptying.

Treatment of Overactive Bladder

toxic effects on the cardiovascular system including lowering of the blood pressure when going from a sitting to standing position (called **orthostatic hypotension**) and abnormal heart rhythms. Thus, it should be kept in a location that is not accessible to younger children. If the patient wishes to discontinue imipramine after a prolonged period of use, it is important to wean off the medication under a doctor's supervision as opposed to stopping it suddenly.

Propiverine. Propiverine is typically given as a 15 mg tablet twice a day. Studies comparing propiverine 15 mg po BID to tolterodine 2 mg po BID demonstrated a similar efficacy between the 2 drugs. The most common side effect of propiverine is dry mouth (20%–47%). Propiverine is not available for use in the United States.

24. What are the side effects of antimuscarinics?

Muscarinic receptors are located throughout the body including the salivary gland, the bowel, and the brain (Figure 5). Thus, an antimuscarinic agent used for the treatment of overactive bladder has the potential of affecting other areas throughout the body. Systemic side effects related to antimuscarinic agents include:

• Dry mouth—The salivary glands contain M1 and M3 receptors, so antimuscarinic agents affect salivary production. Baseline salivary production, that is, the production of saliva at times during the day when one is not eating, is affected by antimuscarinics. It is this constant salivary production that coats our teeth and gums, and maintains our dental health. Saliva is also produced when one eats or drinks something. This eating-induced salivary pro-

---

Orthostatic hypotension

lowering of blood pressure while moving from a sitting to a standing position.

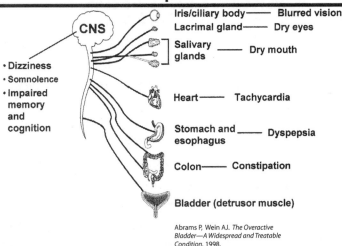

Muscarinic Receptor Distribution

CNS

Iris/ciliary body —— Blurred vision
Lacrimal gland —— Dry eyes
Salivary glands —— Dry mouth

- Dizziness
- Somnolence
- Impaired memory and cognition

Heart —— Tachycardia

Stomach and esophagus —— Dyspepsia

Colon —— Constipation

Bladder (detrusor muscle)

Abrams P, Wein AJ. *The Overactive Bladder—A Widespread and Treatable Condition*, 1998.

Figure 5 Muscarinic receptor locations. (From Abrams P, Wein AJ: The Overactive Bladder: A Widespread and Treatable Condition. Reprinted with permission from Eric Sparre Medical AB.)

duction is not disturbed by antimuscarinics. Dry mouth makes it more difficult to chew and swallow food, makes the oral tissues (gums and tongue) more prone to infection, increases the risk of tooth decay, and makes it more difficult to taste salty, bitter, sweet, and sour flavors.

- Treatments for dry mouth include: frequent sips of water, drinking milk, use of olive oil to moisten your mouth, sugar-free gum and other sugar-free candies, avoiding drinks with caffeine or alcohol, avoiding smoking, and the use of a humidifier at night. Antiseptics may be helpful in keeping the mouth clean and in decreasing the number of bacteria that cause tooth decay and gum disease. Glycerin and lemon mouthwash can be used to try and stimulate saliva production, but these should be used sparingly as too-frequent use can cause tooth decay and gum disease. Use of high concentration fluoride tooth-pastes may also be helpful in preventing tooth decay.

- Constipation—There are muscarinic receptors in the colon (M1 and M3) that govern its ability to contract and propel stool through it. Methods to improve bowel function while on an antimuscarinic include adequate fluid intake, increased fiber intake, and the use of stool softeners and stimulants/laxatives as needed. For those individuals prone to constipation, it is very helpful to get your bowels regular before starting the antimuscarinic therapy.

- Central nervous system—The brain contains muscarinic receptors, but unlike many areas of the body, the brain has a protective barrier: the **blood brain barrier**. This semipermeable barrier prevents a variety of substances, including medications, from entering the brain. Thus, the ability of an antimuscarinic to cause central nervous system side effects is governed by its ability to cross this blood brain barrier and affect a particular receptor. Antimuscarinics that are able to cross the blood brain barrier and affect M1 receptors in the brain may affect one's **cognition** (thinking, learning, and memory). Those antimuscarinic medications that do not affect M1 receptors will not cause problems with cognitive function.

- Urinary retention—Although the antimuscarinics have been shown to decrease uninhibited bladder contractions and increase bladder capacity, they rarely cause urinary retention. In the absence of significant obstruction to the outflow of urine, it does not appear that anticholinergic (antimuscarinic) medications worsen voiding difficulties in women. Studies in women on antimuscarinics have demonstrated no increase in the number of urinary tract

Blood brain barrier (BBB)

semipermeable network of capillaries with special endothelial cells surrounding the brain; the barrier protects the brain from potentially harmful substances.

Cognition

general term encompassing thinking, learning and memory.

infections, no slow stream, and no increase in the amount of urine left in the bladder after voiding (postvoid residual) or changes in the force of urination. In men, antimuscarinics are rarely used alone. Rather, most men are treated with a medication for their prostate, and if symptoms persist and they are emptying their bladder well, then an antimuscarinic medication is added. In this situation, the risk of urinary retention is low.

Side effects of drugs are often a result of the way the drug is administered, is broken down in the body, and its effects on areas in the body other than the bladder.

The use of a several times a day dosing regimen is often associated with high (peak) and low (trough) levels of drug throughout the dosing period. The high levels of drug may be associated with more side effects, whereas the low levels may affect the efficacy of the drug. Thus, the use of a once-a-day preparation, through a sustained release delivery system, allows for a steady amount of drug in the bloodstream throughout the day. This avoidance of peak (high) and trough (low) drug levels helps to decrease the side effects and maximize the benefits of the medication.

Drugs are broken down (metabolized) via different organs in the body. The most common organ involved in drug metabolism is the liver. For a variety of drugs, including many of the drugs used for overactive bladder, the metabolism of the drug by the liver results in a chemical (metabolite) that can also work on overactive bladder, but it can cause side effects that may be similar, worse, or less than the original medication. For those drugs where the metabolite is associated with worse side effects, it is important to develop a way to give the medication to minimize its metabolism by the liver. In doing so, there will be less of the metabolite and more of the original drug around, and thus fewer side effects. There are three ways to accomplish this task. One is to use a slow release capsule that allows for most of the drug to bypass the liver, the second is to use a skin patch, and the third is to place the drug directly into the bladder. All of these ways of administering the drug help to decrease any metabolism by the liver. Lastly, since many organ systems throughout the body have muscarinic receptors, it is important to have a drug that is more selective for the particular organ that is being treated, which is the bladder in the case of overactive bladder. A bladder-selective drug would have a greater effect on the bladder than other organ systems.

25. What is behavioral therapy?

The term **behavioral therapy** encompasses a group of treatment methods that presume that an individual can be educated about his/her medical condition and can develop strategies to minimize or eliminate the symptoms (see Figure 4, in Question 19). For those individuals with overactive bladder, the goals of behavioral therapy are to reduce or eliminate the number of incontinence episodes and the urinary frequency. In individuals with urge incontinence, there is a problem with the bladder and the **pelvic floor muscles**. Thus, behavioral therapy focuses on both the bladder and the pelvic floor muscles. There are several components to behavioral therapy (see Figure 4). Behavioral therapy starts with patient education. The patient must understand normal lower urinary tract anatomy and func-

Behaviorial therapy

a group of treatments designed for educating an individual about his/her medical condition so strategies can be developed to minimize or eliminate the symptoms.

Pelvic floor muscles

a series of muscles that form a sling or hammock across the opening of the pelvis; these muscles, together with their surrounding tissue, are responsible for keeping all of the pelvic organs (bladder, uterus, and rectum) in place and functioning correctly.

tion. Furthermore, the role of the bladder and the pelvic floor muscles in voiding and maintenance of continence must be understood.

Behavioral therapy is often one of the first-line therapies used in the treatment of overactive bladder with or without stress urinary incontinence. It may be combined with pharmacological therapy. Studies assessing the success rates of behavioral therapy and pharmacological therapy demonstrate an improved result with the combination as opposed to either therapy alone.

26. What is the success rate of behavioral therapy?

Although behavioral therapy is effective, it requires motivation and **compliance**. It only works if the exercises are done and the dietary and lifestyle changes are adhered to. For the elderly, there is often the additional need of a dedicated caregiver to assist with therapy. The benefits of behavioral therapy are related to continuation with the therapy. Studies evaluating the durability of behavioral therapy have demonstrated initial response rates of 85% and three-year response rates of 48%. This drop in the response rate is most likely related to a lack of continuation of the behavioral therapy regimen.

Compliance
the consistency and accuracy with which a patient follows the regimen prescribed by a physician or other health care professional.

Patient satisfaction with behavioral therapy for the treatment of overactive bladder with or without stress incontinence is high. This is reflected in the fifth National Association for Continence Survey of 130,000 members, in which 50% of patients ranked conservative therapies in general and 25% ranked pelvic floor muscle exercises specifically as "most helpful."

Physicians have demonstrated an improvement in the frequency of incontinent episodes in 80% of women with urge and mixed incontinence treated with behavioral therapy. In a study, 96.5% of the women were happy to continue with behavioral therapy including pelvic floor muscle exercises indefinitely, and only 14% desired an alternative form of therapy. When compared to oxybutynin, behavioral therapy was associated with a greater percentage reduction in urge incontinence episodes: 84% compared to 72%. Of note, in this study, when behavioral therapy was combined with medical therapy there was an 84.5%–88% reduction in incontinence episodes.

27. What is a voiding diary?

A voiding diary (see Figure 3, in Question 17) is used to help the patient and physician understand the patient's lower urinary tract function. Typically, the doctor will ask that you complete a daily voiding diary over a several day period to assess your symptoms at baseline. The diary also is helpful in the future for evaluating your response to therapy.

The voiding diary has several components. One records the volume voided and the time of each void. In addition, the number and severity of incontinence episodes and the time of such episodes are recorded. The volume of fluid and the type of fluid are also recorded. This allows for identification of those individuals who drink excessive amounts of fluid or who have a high intake of caffeinated fluids.

Caffeine is a diuretic (stimulates the kidneys to produce increased amounts of urine) and a bladder irritant. Those individuals with a high fluid intake, more than 2.5 liters (2.37 quarts) per day, may benefit from decreasing their fluid intake. Similarly, highly acidic diets or overzealous intake of cranberry products, juice, or pills, may lead to an acidic urine that may irritate the bladder. Lastly, poor fluid intake causes the urine to be concentrated and this too may irritate the bladder.

28. What is timed voiding?

Timed voiding is an essential component of behavioral therapy. Typically, one is instructed to void, whether one feels the urge to or not, every two to three hours. For those individuals who suffer from urinary frequency they may already be voiding more frequently than this. For those individuals who suffer from urge incontinence, timed voiding ensures regular emptying of the bladder and ideally will decrease the volume of urine that is lost at the time of an urge incontinent episode. In the elderly, a caregiver will be required to prompt voiding and assist the individual with getting to and from the bathroom.

Timed voiding
a type of therapy that involves urinating at two- to three-hour intervals, no matter if there is an urge

Those individuals who suffer from urgency and frequency without urge incontinence can try to delay voiding. With delayed voiding, the individual consciously tries to ignore the urge sensation and hold his/her urine for a progressively longer period of time to gradually increase his/her bladder capacity.

29. What are pelvic floor muscle exercises or Kegel exercises?

Developed in 1948 by Dr. Arnold Kegel, this series of exercises involve the pelvic floor muscles. Pelvic floor muscles are a group of muscles that are attached to the

Kegel exercises
exercises designed to strengthen weak pelvic floor muscles.

pelvic bone and act like a hammock to support the pelvic organs, which include the bladder, uterus, and rectum. These muscles may be weakened by childbirth, prior pelvic surgery, or obesity. Kegel exercises have been used in the treatment of stress urinary incontinence since the late 1940s with cure rates up to 84% reported.

The use of pelvic floor muscle exercises in the treatment of pure urge incontinence and mixed urinary incontinence (urge incontinence plus stress incontinence) is based on the observations that contraction (tightening) of the pelvic floor muscles inhibits detrusor contractions. Pelvic floor muscle exercises require a motivated, diligent, and properly instructed individual. Similar to weight lifting, strengthening of the pelvic floor muscles requires repetitive contractions of the pelvic floor muscles on a daily basis. Infrequent performance will not lead to beneficial results.

Most people find it difficult to identify the pelvic floor muscles and to contract these muscles. Typically, when an individual is asked to contract the pelvic floor muscles, the muscles of the buttocks are tightened. Actually, neither the buttock nor the thigh muscles are involved in these exercises. Placing a finger or special weight (called a vaginal cone) in the vagina (for women) or anus (for men) and contracting the muscles will produce a tightening around the finger or prevent loss of the weight if the person is in a standing position. Both are helpful strategies to identify the pelvic floor muscles. For those individuals who have a difficult time identifying the pelvic floor muscles, biofeedback can be used to identify them (see Question 32).

A good way to start Kegel exercises is to perform the exercises for five minutes twice a day. You should tighten/squeeze the pelvic floor muscles for a count of 4, and then relax for a count of 4, doing this repetitively for a total of five minutes. If you find that you cannot do this for a full five minutes at the start, then decrease to a tolerable time and gradually build up to five minutes. The exercises can be done anytime and anywhere. It is easiest to perform the exercises at the same times each day to help build a routine.

30. How successful are Kegel exercises?

Kathy's comment:

I tried Kegel exercises without success for the stress incontinence, however, I was having some urge incontinence. I did notice an improvement with the urge incontinence slowly after about 3–4 months.

The results of Kegel exercises will not occur immediately. Similar to weight lifting, it takes time to strengthen the pelvic floor muscles and they will only remain strong when one is regularly performing the exercises. In most women, it will take 6 to 12 weeks to notice a change in urine loss, provided that the exercises are being performed properly and regularly. Several studies have confirmed the efficacy of pelvic floor muscle exercises in urge and mixed urinary incontinence. In one clinical study, the number of urge incontinence episodes per week decreased by 80%, and the time between voiding increased from 2.13 hours to 3.44 hours with the use of pelvic floor muscle exercises.

31. Who is a candidate for Kegel exercises?

Kathy's comment:

Almost anyone is a candidate for these type of exercises. This is especially true if you leak urine. My experience is a little bit out of the ordinary. As a nurse, I have taught patients how to do Kegel exercises which allowed me to utilize the technique efficiently as soon as I started. Nevertheless, it was clear to me early on that you have to be very dedicated and extremely motivated to achieve success. Finally, it is important to realize that these exercises are for long term.

The ideal candidate for Kegel exercises is a highly motivated individual. This person must be capable of learning the exercises and performing the exercises on his or her own. To facilitate learning the individual must be able to understand and follow directions. In addition, he/she must realize that Kegel exercises require a commitment to long-term therapy. Kegel exercises are effective in stress, urge, and mixed urinary incontinence, and thus in the absence of motivational and educational factors virtually everyone is a candidate for Kegel exercises.

Biofeedback

information about one or more of an individual's normally unconscious body processes is made available to the individual through a visual (see), auditory (hear), or tactile (touch) signal.

32. What is biofeedback?

Biofeedback is a form of learning and re-education. With biofeedback information about one or more of an individual's normally unconscious normal body processes is made available to the individual through a visual (see), auditory (hear), or tactile (touch) signal. Objective responses can be recorded on a tracing so the individual can review them.

When evaluating pelvic floor muscle activity, an electromyography is performed whereas a cystometrogram is used to measure and evaluate bladder muscle activity. Electromyography measures the activity of select muscles by the use of electrodes that are placed near or into the muscles. To evaluate the pelvic floor muscles, the electrodes may be placed on the skin near the anus, or special probes may be placed into the vagina, anus or urethra. These electrodes are connected to a specialized machine that displays the activity of the muscles on a screen and records it onto a paper tracing. Relaxation of the pelvic floor muscles leads to a flat line on the tracing whereas contraction of the muscles leads to an up-and-down line on the tracing. The patient is then able to see when he/she is relaxing or contracting the pelvic floor muscles.

33. Who is a candidate for biofeedback?

Not all individuals will need biofeedback. Those individuals who are having trouble identifying their pelvic floor muscles or who are failing pelvic floor muscle exercises are candidates for biofeedback. As with pelvic floor muscle exercises, biofeedback requires a highly motivated individual who performs the exercises daily.

34. What is the success rate of biofeedback?

The combination of behavioral therapy including Kegel exercises and biofeedback has been shown to be superior to either therapy alone. This form of therapy works better for stress urinary incontinence than urge incontinence, however. Younger women and those without estrogen deficiency tend to do better with biofeedback than older women and women with low estrogen levels.

35. What are capsaicin and resiniferatoxin?

Capsaicin is the active ingredient found in chili peppers. **Resiniferatoxin** is a chemical derived from a cactus-like plant, *Euphorbia resinifera*. Resiniferatoxin is roughly 100 times more potent than capsaicin. How hot are these chemicals? The spice industry uses a scale, called the Scoville scale, to compare pepper strengths in heat units. Bell peppers are barely a 1 on the Scoville scale, whereas pure capsaicin has a score of 16 million and resiniferatoxin a score of 16 billion Scoville heat units. Thus, both capsaicin and resiniferatoxin are very hot.

36. How do capsaicin and resiniferatoxin work?

Inside the bladder there are two types of nerves that travel from the bladder to the central nervous system. These nerves are responsible for transmitting signals of fullness and/or discomfort from the bladder to the brain. One type of nerve, the small A delta fiber, transmits signals regarding bladder fullness, and nerves called C fibers detect noxious signals and initiate painful sensations. C fibers are typically excited when there is an irritation and/or infection of the bladder. When stimulated, these C fibers can facilitate or cause voiding.

When placed into the bladder, both capsaicin and resiniferatoxin cause an intense stimulation of the C fibers. This intense stimulation causes the nerves to run out of neurotransmitters, so they cannot transmit messages to the brain and spinal cord that would cause the bladder to contract. Because there is no permanent damage to the nerves, the therapy is not permanent.

However, it does take the nerves a fair amount of time to build up a new supply of neurotransmitters.

When placed into the bladder of an awake individual with normal sensation, capsaicin causes significant discomfort. In fact, it is far too uncomfortable to do this procedure without the use of either a general or spinal anesthesia. Resiniferatoxin, although it is more potent than capsaicin, does not require anesthesia because there is no intense pain when it is placed into the bladder.

37. How effective are capsaicin and resiniferatoxin? How are they administered and how long will the response last?

In a review of several studies using capsaicin to treat overactive bladder from a variety of causes, it appeared that capsaicin was effective in decreasing bladder overactivity. Studies showed that it was more effective in individuals with overactive bladder from a neurogenic cause, such as that related to a spinal cord injury, multiple sclerosis, myelomeningocele, etc. It is less effective in individuals with overactive bladder of a nonneurologic cause, that is, those with hypersensitive bladders and individuals with pelvic pain. Clinical studies with resiniferatoxin suggest that it produces clinical improvement in individuals with overactive bladder of both neurologic and nonneurologic causes.

The effect of capsaicin may not be immediate. In fact, it may take up to two months for an improvement to occur. Some individuals may notice a transient worsening of their symptoms, which may last for one to two weeks and then disappear. But those individuals who note an improvement in their bladder symptoms with capsaicin find that the response lasts anywhere from three to six months to over one year.

Most of the studies using resiniferatoxin have been short-term studies. Unlike capsaicin, there did not appear to be a transient worsening of the patient's symptoms after resiniferatoxin instillation. With resiniferatoxin, the results were often noted as soon as one day after the treatment, and in those who responded the response lasted for at least three months, the longest time that was evaluated.

Neither capsaicin nor resiniferatoxin are currently approved for routine clinical intravesical use. These medications should be administered by a physician who is familiar with their use and who has achieved the approval of the local institutional review board and regulatory authorities.

Capsaicin administration may be performed in the clinic in those individuals who have no bladder sensation, such as those with a spinal cord injury. Otherwise, it is typically instilled under general anesthesia. A dose of 50 to 100 milliliters (ml) of 1 to 2 mM (millimolar) capsaicin dissolved in 30% ethanol in saline is the dose most commonly used for overactive bladder. A catheter is placed into the bladder, the urine is drained, and then the capsaicin is administered. The capsaicin is left in the bladder for approximately 30 minutes and then is drained out.

Resiniferatoxin does not cause the bladder pain that capsaicin does and, thus, it can be administered in the clinic. Since resiniferatoxin is much more potent than capsaicin, a lower dose can be used. The recommended concentration of resiniferatoxin is not yet clearly defined. Studies have used concentrations that have ranged from 1 nM (nanomole) to 10 μM (micromole). Resiniferatoxin is usually dissolved in 10% ethanol and is placed into the bladder in a similar volume and duration as capsaicin.

38. What are the side effects of capsaicin and resiniferatoxin?

Temporary worsening of urinary symptoms can occur for a few weeks after capsaicin use. Symptoms may include suprapubic (above the pubic bone) and perineal (relating to the perineum) pain, burning sensation, urinary frequency, urinary incontinence, and hematuria (presence of red blood cells in the urine). Urinary tract infections may occur as a result of **catheterization** with either capsaicin or resiniferatoxin use. If the capsaicin or resiniferatoxin leaks onto the skin, it may cause local skin irritation.

In those individuals with a spinal cord injury and a condition called autonomic dysreflexia, there is a risk of causing **hypertension**. These individuals should have the procedure performed under anesthesia with continuous blood pressure monitoring. These individuals should be monitored closely and have a Foley catheter for several days after the procedure.

MINIMALLY INVASIVE OPTIONS

39. What is botulinum toxin?

Botulinum neurotoxin is one of the most poisonous biological chemicals known. It is a chemical that is produced by the bacterium *Clostridium botulinum*. Very

Catheterization

a tubular instrument especially designed to be passed through the urethra and drain it of retained urine.

Hypertension

transitory or sustained elevated arterial blood pressure.

Botulinum neurotoxin

a poisonous biological chemical produced by the bacterium *Clostridium botulinum* that is used medically to cause temporary muscle paralysis.

small amounts of botulinum toxin can lead to paralysis. This may result from clostridial infection of the intestines, a wound, or eating food that is contaminated by *Clostridium botulinum*. The *Clostridium botulinum* bacteria produce a variety of types of botulinum toxin. The toxin that is used most commonly in medicine is the botulinum toxin-A type. All of the different types of botulinum toxin produce a weakening and lack of activity of the affected muscles.

40. How does botulinum toxin work in overactive bladder?

Botulinum has been shown to prevent the release of the neurotransmitter, acetylcholine, from parasympathetic and cholinergic nerves. In the case of an overactive bladder, it is the release of acetylcholine from the parasympathetic neuron that results in the stimulus for the bladder muscle to contract. When the release of acetylcholine is prevented, there is no stimulus for bladder muscle contraction. For the toxin to be effective it must be injected directly into the bladder muscle. The bladder is readily accessible through the **cystoscope**. The cystoscope, a long telescope-like instrument, is passed through the urethra into the bladder. After inspection of the bladder, the bladder muscle is injected with the botulinum toxin through a slender hollow needle that is passed through the cystoscope into the wall of the bladder. Because the toxin only works locally and does not diffuse through the muscle of the bladder, multiple injections, typically in the range of 30 to 40, using very small amounts of the toxin, are performed during the procedure.

The botulinum toxin does not produce a permanent change in the bladder muscle and typically its effects

Cystoscope

a long telescope-like instrument that is passed through the urethra into the bladder for diagnostic and therapeutic purposes.

will last for around three months. Therefore, patients often need repeat injections over the course of time.

41. How effective is botulinum toxin in overactive bladder?

Botulinum toxin bladder injection has been safely used in individuals with overactive bladder as a result of spinal cord injury who have failed maximal medical therapy. In such individuals, an improvement in the number of incontinence episodes and on the bladder pressures was noted in the majority of patients. The toxin appeared to decrease the bladder contractility for at least nine months from the injection. At present, botulinum toxin is being used for those individuals with overactive bladder from non-neurologic causes that are refractory (that is, resistant to treatment) to all other medical therapies.

42. What are the side effects of the botulinum toxin?

Injections with botulinum toxin are usually well tolerated. Once injected, the toxin diffuses into the surrounding muscle and surrounding tissues, but its effect decreases with increasing distance from the injection site. If the injection goes beyond the bladder wall, then there may be an effect on muscles and tissue outside of the bladder.

Rarely, the injection of the toxin will be associated with a flu-like illness. Botulinum toxin should not be used in a pregnant woman or a woman who is breast-feeding. The effects of botulinum toxin in children are not well known. The cystoscopy itself and injections may cause a temporary irritation to the urethra and bladder, leading to short-term discomfort with urination (dysuria) and blood in the urine (hematuria). Rarely, an individual can develop a urinary tract infection. The long-term effects of botulinum toxin on the bladder muscle are not well known.

43. What is neuromodulation/sacral nerve stimulation?

Neuromodulation

surgical placement of a permanent continuous nerve stimulator and its electrode wires.

Neuromodulation using the device, Interstim Continence Control System (Medtronic, Inc,. Minneapolis, MN), is a form of electrical stimulation that was approved by the FDA in 1997. It has been used throughout Europe since 1994. The technique involves the surgical placement of a permanent continuous nerve stimulator and its electrode wires (Figure 6).

The mechanism by which sacral nerve stimulation affects bladder dysfunction is not entirely understood. One theory is that urgency and urge incontinence may be associated with dysfunction of the pelvic floor muscles and the urethral sphincter muscles. It is thought that by stimulation of the sacral nerves, particularly the pelvic and pudendal nerves, the "stimulated" nerves will decrease the "spastic" activity of the pelvic floor muscles and increase the tone of the urethral sphincter. In addition, it is thought that stimulation of certain nerves including sensory nerves in the pelvic floor may lead to inhibition of the nerves that stimulate the bladder to contract.

44. Who is a candidate for sacral neuromodulation?

Candidates for sacral neuromodulation are those individuals who have failed first-line therapies including behavioral therapy and oral therapy. Sacral neuromodulation

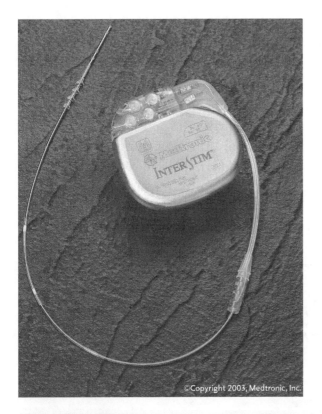

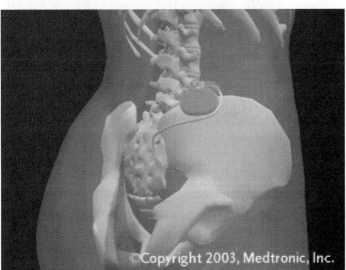

Figure 6   Neuromodulation device. A) Neurostim device. B) Placement of the Neurostim device. (Reprinted with permission from Medtronic, Inc. © 2004).

may be considered before invasive surgical procedures such as urinary diversion and bladder augmentation.

All individuals considering sacral neuromodulation should undergo a complete urologic and neurologic evaluation. This evaluation should include: a history; physical examination; urinalysis; radiologic evaluation of the kidneys, bladder, and lower spinal column including the **sacrum**; a urodynamic study; and a cystoscopy. This extensive evaluation is to ensure that there are no other conditions present that may cause or mimic the overactive bladder symptoms, such as bladder cancer, urinary tract infections, etc.

Sacrum

refers to the large, irregular, triangular shaped bone made up of the five fused vertebrae below the lumbar region; comprises the pelvis.

45. How is sacral neuromodulation performed?

There are three stages to the implantation of the Interstim device.

- Phase 1—To identify the proper location of the sacral nerves.
- Phase 2—Placement of external wires to test the individual's response to the electrical stimulation.
- Phase 3—Implantation of the Interstim device (Figure 7, in Question 43).

Phase 1

This phase may be performed with the patient under local or general anesthesia. The patient is placed in a prone (lying facedown) position. The sacrum is palpated to feel for the openings (foramina) in the sacrum. Two needle electrodes, one on each side, are placed into the sacral foramina. Stimulating the electrodes and evaluating the response confirm the proper positioning of the electrodes. If the electrodes are in the proper position, the pelvic floor muscles will contract with stimulation of the needle electrode and the big toe will bend. If the needle electrodes are not in the correct position, they are repositioned until they are in the proper place. Phase 1 may be combined with Phase 2 in the same procedure.

Phase 2

Once the correct position of the needle electrodes is confirmed, external stimulation wires replace them. The wires may be taped in place or tunneled under the skin to prevent them from falling out over the following three- to four-day test period. The external wires are connected to a portable hand-held neurostimulator. The patient is discharged to home the same day and is asked to complete a **micturition** (voiding) diary over the following three to four days. A urodynamic study is obtained prior to the fourth day to assess the patient's response. A positive response is an improvement in clinical symptoms by at least 50%. At the end of the three to four days the wires are removed.

Phase 3

Those patients who responded positively during the trial with the external stimulation wires are candidates for implantation of the permanent device. Typically, there is at least a two-week interval between removal of the external stimulation wires and placement of the permanent device, to decrease the chance of developing an infection. This procedure is performed under general anesthesia. One or, more commonly, two (one on each side) permanent electrodes are placed into the sacral canal via the third sacral foramina in the pelvis. To prevent movement of the electrode it is secured in place. The wires are tunneled under the skin to bring

Treatment of Overactive Bladder

Micturition

the act of voiding urine.

them to the stimulating device, which is placed under the skin in the groin area.

46. What is the success rate of sacral neuromodulation?

Of those individuals with refractory (resistant to treatment) urge incontinence, only about 50% will have a positive response to the test stimulation. In those who have a positive response with test stimulation and who undergo permanent implantation, there is a durable positive result for at least five years in about 60% of the individuals.

Studies in women with an average age between 43 and 50 years demonstrated that about 40% of the women remained dry over the long term and the remainder noted a more than 50% improvement in their urge incontinent episodes. A study of 25 patients older than 55 years of age with refractory urge incontinence demonstrated that 25 (48%) had a positive response to the test stimulation. After implantation of the permanent device, all 25 noted a more than 50% reduction in their urge incontinent episodes and two individuals became totally dry.

In another study, 51 patients with refractory urge incontinence and a positive response to phase 2 were randomized to either a control group or a stimulation group. Compared to the control group, the stimulation group demonstrated statistically significant improvements with respect to the number of voids daily, volume voided, and the degree of urgency. In addition, the stimulation group demonstrated statistically significant improvements in quality of life when compared to the control group.

Individuals who do not tend to respond as well to Interstim include male patients with refractory urge incontinence and those individuals whose first unstable bladder contraction occurs at a small bladder volume. The latter underscores the need for urodynamic studies prior to performing the procedure. Lastly, individuals with significant psychological or psychiatric problems with overactive bladder tend to fail therapy more often that individuals without psychological problems.

47. What are the risks of placement of a sacral neuromodulation device?

The complication rate associated with placement of a permanent sacral neuromodulation device is low. Overall, the complication rate is 22%–43% with a reoperation rate of 6%–50%. Complications may be related to the surgical procedure or to the function of the device.

Surgical related complications include:

- Discomfort related to placement and tunneling of the electrode wires and the neurostimulator device.
- Wound infections and infections around the neurostimulator device.
- Migration of the electrodes.

Complications related to the device itself include:

- Uncomfortable sensations related to too high of an electrical current.
- Broken electrodes.
- Mechanical problems with the device.
- Battery exhaustion.

Treatment of Overactive Bladder

48. Are there other forms of electrical stimulation besides sacral nerve stimulation?

Yes, there are other forms of electrical stimulation that have been used to treat a variety of voiding troubles. Pelvic floor electrostimulation has been used to strengthen the sphincter, the muscles around the urethra, and the pelvic floor muscles. These forms of stimulation may be **transcutaneous** by placing the stimulator device on the skin in the appropriate area. Electrical stimulation has been shown to increase bladder capacity. It has also been used for stress urinary incontinence. Few studies are available regarding the success and durability of this type of therapy.

Transcutaneous

denotes the passage of substances through the unbroken skin.

SURGICAL OPTIONS

49. What is bladder augmentation?

Bladder augmentation is a surgical procedure whereby the bladder is enlarged. The increase in size may be by the addition of other tissues, such as a segment of intestine, a segment of the stomach, or utilization of a segment of dilated ureter (Figure 7). In addition, the bladder may be enlarged functionally by removing the detrusor muscle from the bladder lining, called the **mucosa**. The goals of bladder augmentation are to:

Bladder augmentation

a surgical procedure whereby the bladder is enlarged.

Mucosa

a mucous tissue lining various tubular structures, including the bladder.

- Enable storage of urine at a low bladder pressure.
- Help the patient achieve continence.
- Avoid damage to the kidneys.
- Allow the patient to empty his/her bladder in a timely and convenient manner.

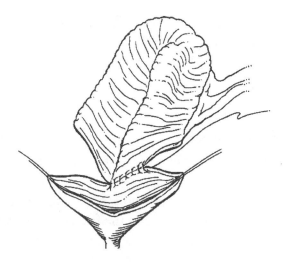

Figure 7   Bladder augmentation.

50. Who is a candidate for bladder augmentation?

Bladder augmentation is not considered a first-line therapy for the management of overactive bladder. In fact, it is considered only when all other methods of treatment have failed. Individuals who are undergoing bladder augmentation must be willing to take the risk that they will be dependent on **clean intermittent catheterization** (CIC) to empty their bladder for the rest of their life. Most people can learn how to perform this procedure. First, the patient must learn his or her own urological anatomy. He or she also must be able to reach the urethra and learn how to manipulate the catheter (tube) to empty the bladder properly.

Candidates should also be aware of the permanent nature of the procedure and the risks related to the type of bladder augmentation being performed. Those individuals with small bladder capacities, with elevated

Clean intermittent catheterization

a type of temporary catheter to remove urine from the body; usually self-accomplished by inserting the tube through the urethra to empty the bladder.

bladder pressures, and uninhibited bladder contractions with normal urethral sphincter function are the best candidates for bladder augmentation.

51. What are the types of bladder augmentation?

There are several different ways to enlarge the bladder including enterocystoplasty, gastrocystoplasty, autoaugmentation, and ureterocystoplasty. There are studies being performed to determine the feasibility of growing cells in the laboratory to use for bladder augmentation.

Enterocystoplasty—Enterocystoplasty is the most common method for bladder augmentation. It is the procedure to which all other bladder enlargement procedures are compared. With enterocystoplasty, the bladder is made larger by the addition of a segment of small or large intestine. Traditionally, the ileum, which is a segment of the small intestine, is used. The piece of intestine is isolated from the remainder of the intestine and the continuity of the remaining intestine re-established. The isolated piece of intestine is then opened and reconfigured as a patch. It is important that the intestinal piece is opened and reconfigured, since leaving it in its normal shape as a tube would allow it to retain its normal ability to contract and relax. Doing that would lead to increased bladder pressures, the opposite of the desired action. The surgery is performed under general anesthesia. Typically it is performed through a midline abdominal cut (**incision**); however, some urologists are performing all or part of the procedure **laparoscopically**. The bladder is opened either longitudinally or it may be opened both longitu-

Enterocystoplasty

a surgical procedure to enlarge the bladder by the addition of a segment of small or large intestine.

Incision

a cut, a surgical wound.

Laparoscopic

type of microsurgery using a tiny laparoscope passed through the skin and into the organ, with a fiberoptic camera and surgical tools inserted to view and perform the surgery.

dinally and transversely. It is important that the bladder be opened fully, as this helps prevent unstable bladder contractions and increases in bladder pressure after the procedure. The intestinal patch is then sewn to the bladder. Typically, a drainage tube, called a Foley catheter or a suprapubic tube, is left in place for at least a week to allow for healing. The hospital stay is usually around five to seven days, depending on when bowel function returns. A **cystogram**, a study in which contrast material is inserted through the drainage tube into the bladder and x-rays obtained, is performed to rule out any leaks prior to the tube removal.

Advantages of enterocystoplasty include:

- The presence of adequate amounts of intestine in most individuals.
- Long-term success rates; 77% of patients with intractable overactive bladder are voiding and continent with ileal enterocystoplasty.
- Increases in bladder capacity.

Disadvantages of enterocystoplasty include:

- Early complications related to enterocystoplasty include: bleeding, infection, urinary leakage, and wound breakdown.
- Late complications related to enterocystoplasty include: intra-abdominal adhesions leading to a bowel obstruction, urinary tract infections, bladder and kidney stones, and bladder rupture.
- Production of mucus by the bowel segment requires bladder irrigation to prevent obstruction, infections, and stone formation.

Treatment of Overactive Bladder

Cystogram
a type of test where fluid called contrast material is inserted through the drainage tube into the bladder and x-rays are obtained. The contrast material causes specific areas of the body to be "lit up" by the x-rays, so that the radiologist can analyze the area.

- Long-term risk of malignancy; this is rare and in the few patients who developed a cancer, it was identified 15 years or more after the augmentation. Because of this risk it is recommended that periodic surveillance with a cystoscopy and a **urine cytology** be performed. To perform a urine cytology, a small amount of urine is sent to a pathologist, who examines the urine to determine the presence or absence of any cancer cells in the urine.

- Although some individuals may be able to void spontaneously after bladder augmentation, all patients must be prepared to perform life-long clean intermittent catheterization (see Question 50).

- Electrolyte abnormalities are common with enterocystoplasty. The isolated segment of intestine continues to function like a normal intestine. It is able to absorb certain chemicals in the urine. Because of this absorption of chemicals from the urine, periodic blood testing is required. Some individuals will require the addition of medications to counteract the acid that is reabsorbed by the intestinal segment.

Gastrocystoplasty—Gastrocystoplasty is similar to enterocystoplasty, except that instead of using a piece of intestine, a segment of the stomach is used to patch the bladder. This procedure has been more commonly used in children with overactive bladder from a neurologic abnormality. As with enterocystoplasty, the procedure requires entry into the abdominal cavity and involves the isolation of a segment of the stomach with closure of the stomach defect. This segment of stomach does not require reconfiguration, as it is not tube

---

Urine cytology

a small amount of urine is sent to the pathologist, who examines the urine sample to determine the presence or absence of any cancer cells.

Gastrocystoplasty

similar to enterocystoplasty, except that instead of using a piece of intestine, a segment of the stomach is used to patch the bladder.

shaped. The segment of stomach is then sewn as a "patch" to the opened bladder.

Advantages of gastrocystoplasty include:

- The stomach does not produce mucus, so the risk of infections and stones is far less. Since there is no mucus production, the augmented bladder does not require irrigation.
- The risk of long-term malignancy may be decreased by using the stomach instead of the small intestine for aumentation.
- The risk of obstruction where the continuity of the stomach was re-established is lower than enterocystoplasty (with the intestine).
- Electrolyte abnormalities are less severe with stomach than intestinal patches and less commonly require medical treatment.

Disadvantages of gastrocystoplasty include:

- The stomach patch continues to produce acid, and this may lead acidic urine that irritates the tissues and causes discomfort with urination (dysuria) and blood in the urine (hematuria).
- There needs to be adequate length of the blood supply to the stomach segment to allow the stomach patch to move from the upper abdomen down into the pelvis.

Autoaugmentation—Autoaugmentation is the surgical procedure in which a part of the bladder muscle—the detrusor—is removed from the bladder. By removing the detrusor from a segment of the bladder, the ability of that segment to contract is destroyed.

Autoaugmentation

a surgical procedure in which a part of the bladder muscle—the detrusor—is removed from the bladder.

Since the procedure requires access only to the bladder, the surgery does not require entry into the abdominal cavity, only the pelvis.

Advantages of autoaugmentation include:

- Less invasive procedure than enterocystoplasty.
- No risk of bowel obstruction.
- Faster recovery than enterocystoplasty.
- Effective in decreasing uninhibited bladder contractions.

Disadvantages of autoaugmentation include:

- Lack of consistent improvement in bladder capacity.
- May require clean intermittent catheterization for bladder emptying (see Question 50).

Ureterocystoplasty—Ureterocystoplasty is a technique used in patients who have a dilated distal ureter, which can be isolated, opened, and used as a bladder patch.

Ureterocystoplasty
technique is used in patients who have a dilated distal ureter, which can be isolated, opened, and used as a bladder patch.

Advantages of ureterocystoplasty include:

- Use of native urothelial tissue, which behaves like the normal tissue lining the bladder and, thus, there is no mucus production.
- Does not require entry into the abdominal cavity and, thus, there is no risk of a bowel obstruction or bowel adhesions.

Disadvantages of ureterocystoplasty include:

Vesicoureteral reflux
urine passing backwards from the bladder to the kidney.

- It cannot be used in most patients because it requires that the individual has a dilated ureter, which is not common. Candidates for this procedure are those with high grade **vesicoureteral reflux** (urine passing backwards from the bladder to the kidney) or those with an obstructed distal ureter. Typically, this procedure is performed in infants who are born with structural abnormalities that cause the ureter to dilate.

- Requires either removal of the ipsilateral kidney or a simultaneous procedure to establish drainage of the kidney. When the distal ureter is separated from the proximal ureter, the proximal ureter needs to be reconnected to the bladder or to the ureter on the opposite side of the body; this permits the urine from the kidney to drain out of the kidney and into the bladder. If this cannot be done or the kidney is not functioning, then the kidney needs to be removed.

- Although it appears that those individuals who are voiding on their own and who undergo ureterocystoplasty have a greater likelihood of being able to void on their own after the surgery, there is still the chance that the bladder will not empty adequately. That would require long-term, clean intermittent catheterization for bladder emptying.

Other techniques now being investigated

Animal studies have shown that it is possible to make the ureter dilate over time, and when the ureter is adequately dilated, a ureterocystoplasty can be performed. This procedure has not been done yet in humans, however. It would carry the same advantages of a straightforward ureterocystoplasty, but would require additional time and an additional procedure to dilate the normal ureter.

Since many of the problems related to enterocystoplasty are due to the ability of the lining of the intestine to release (secrete) and take up (reabsorb) chemicals in the urine, basic scientists and urologists have looked at whether the lining of the intestine could be removed and used as a patch. This preliminary technique has been used in a few humans, but the numbers of patients who have undergone this procedure are too small to make any strong conclusions and long-term information is limited.

Tissue engineering

a pioneering technique of growing cells designed to mimic the behavior and reproducibility of normal cells.

Research currently is focused on **tissue engineering** of bladders using cell transplantation. This is an exciting area of research, since theoretically it would allow a few cells from an individual's bladder to be removed and grown in the proper laboratory setting in sheets, so that the different layers of the bladder develop. These sheets of cells could then be transplanted directly into the bladder. This might be the ideal technique for bladder augmentation, but it is still in the experimental stages and will require much more testing before it can be used in humans.

52. What are bladder denervation procedures?

Bladder denervation procedures are designed to interrupt the nerve supply to the bladder. By interrupting the nerves that stimulate the bladder muscle to contract, it can prevent bladder contractions. If the sensory fibers in the bladder are interrupted, then this may also prevent bladder contractions because it prevents the bladder from sending messages to the central nervous system. Since neurologic control of bladder function occurs centrally (in the brain and spinal column), peripherally, and within the bladder itself, new techniques have focused on interrupting cell signaling in these areas. These procedures may be reversible or irreversible (permanent).

Reversible procedures

The simplest form of bladder denervation is **mucosal anesthesia**. An anesthetic agent is placed into the urethra, bladder, or rectum. This will only affect the sensory fibers. In theory, if the patient responds to this procedure, it would confirm that the problem is one of bladder sensation stimulating the overactivity.

Local anesthesia can be injected into the sacrum to block the sacral nerves supplying the bladder. Alternatively a spinal anesthetic can be administered.

Mucosal anesthesia
a type of procedure still being studied where an anesthetic agent is placed into the urethra, bladder, or rectum, to affect the sensory fibers in the bladder.

Irreversible procedures

In individuals with an overactive bladder secondary to spinal cord injury, specialized spinal surgery to interrupt the nerves stimulating the bladder has been effective. However, after this procedure the bladder fails to contract, and the patient must empty his/her bladder by **clean intermittent catheterization**.

In females with refractory overactive bladder, a transvaginal procedure called the **Ingelman-Sundberg procedure** has been used. Prior to surgery the nerves that would be denervated by the procedure are injected with a local anesthetic. If the woman notes an improvement in her symptoms, then the procedure is carried out. This procedure is not used often and thus results on only a small number of patients are available. In a series of 25 women who underwent the Ingelman-Sundberg procedure for uninhibited bladder contractions, 64% became dry, 8% had temporary improvement in their symptoms, and 28% reported no change in their incontinence episodes.

Ingelman-Sundberg procedure
a transvaginal surgical technique that denerves the bladder to achieve control over uninhibited bladder contractions.

PART FOUR

Diagnosis and Treatment of Stress Urinary Incontinence

What are the different types of SUI, and how are they different?

What is a urodynamic study?

What are the surgical options for women with SUI?

What is an in situ vaginal wall sling?

More ...

53. What is stress urinary incontinence?

Stress urinary incontinence, which is also known as genuine stress urinary incontinence (GSUI), is the involuntary loss of bladder control during periods of increased abdominal pressure such as coughing, laughing, or straining. Normally, the bladder and the first part of the urethra, the tube that one urinates through, are supported by muscles in the pelvis. When these muscles are weakened, there is a lack of support in the bladder, which can lead to the first part of the urethra, the proximal uretha, "drops" (descends) out of the pelvis into the vagina in women. The result of this descent is an unequal distribution of pressure to the bladder and urethra during coughs, laughs, or sneezes. In individuals with normal support who cough, laugh, or sneeze, that increase in pressure is transmitted to both the bladder and the first portion of the urethra. Thus, the pressure remains the same. However, when there are weakened pelvic floor muscles the first part of the urethra and the lower part of the bladder descends out of the pelvis and the increase in pressure is transmitted only to the bladder. Therefore, the bladder pressure overpowers the urethral pressure and leakage occurs. In a unique form of stress incontinence, named Type III stress incontinence, the problem is not a result of weakened pelvis floor muscles; rather, it is a problem with the urethra itself. In this type of incontinence, the urethra itself doesn't close, so any increase in bladder pressure overpowers the urethra.

Stress urinary incontinence (SUI) is a distressing symptom and it may have a major impact on a woman's quality of life. Although it can affect women of all ages, most commonly it affects women between the ages of 20 and 65. Shockingly, over 20% of women are affected in this age group. This problem affects millions of women at a cost of billions of US health care dollars. Stress urinary incontinence is one of the top 20 chronic conditions in the United States.

In answer to a questionnaire asking how symptoms of SUI affect her life, one patient commented:

The symptoms were insidious. They developed slowly but continued to become more progressive and disturbing. At first, I noticed a small amount of leakage when I went jogging. At first I could deal with it but as time went on the symptoms became increasingly more annoying and every day I would wear a panty liner because I feared having an accident. Soon, sneezing and laughing also resulted in leakage. Eventually, I got to the point where I was wearing a pad on a daily basis because the leakage had progressed to the point that I feared soaking though a panty liner.

54. What are the different types of SUI and how do they differ?

Typically, SUI is divided into those types that are related to increased mobility of the urethra and those that are related to poor closure of the urethra. On clinical examination, with a Valsalva maneuver (straining) the urethra is noted to move (hypermobility) and leakage is often noted. However, it is the **Valsalva leak point pressure** (see Question 58) that is used to delineate urethral hypermobility–related SUI from that of poor closure of the urethra (internal sphincter dysfunction). The Valsalva leak point pressure is the intra-abdominal pressure generated by a Valsalva maneuver

Valsalva leak point pressure

the intra-abdominal pressure generated by a Valsalva maneuver that results in urinary leakage.

that results in urinary leakage. This pressure is measured during a urodynamic evaluation for SUI (see Question 58). With hypermobility of the urethra, the Valsalva leak point pressure is high, typically at pressures greater than 60, and often 120 to 130 cm water (H_2O). With poor urethral closure, Type III stress incontinence, the Valsalva leak point pressure is low, and may be as low as 5 cm H_2O.

There is a new device, Monitorr (produced by Johnson & Johnson Company), which measures a parameter called the **urethral resistance profile (URP)** that has been shown to correlate with the type of SUI. This is easier to perform and may be done in the office over a five-minute period.

Urethral resistance profile (URP)

measurement used in urodynamic studies to determine the strength of the urethra.

55. Is stress urinary incontinence a natural result of aging? Who is at risk for developing stress urinary incontinence?

The concept that stress urinary incontinence (SUI) is a natural result of aging is a myth. It is true that the risk of developing stress urinary incontinence increases with age, but it is not inevitable that as you age you will develop SUI. There are a variety of factors that can increase one's risk of developing SUI. The most significant risk factor is multiple childbirths via vaginal delivery. Pregnancy and vaginal delivery can significantly stretch and actually tear the muscles that support the bladder and proximal urethra, such that after delivery and healing they are unable to regain their prior strength. These weakened muscles provide little support to the bladder and proximal urethra. A woman's hormonal status also contributes to the health of these muscles, and postmenopausal women tend to have less healthy vaginal, urethral, and surrounding tissues.

Other causes of pelvic floor weakness include:

- **Congenital** (existing at birth, hereditary).
- Traumatic causes other than labor, such as a pelvic fracture or prior pelvic surgery.
- Inflammatory conditions, such as **pelvic inflammatory disease (PID)**.
- Chronic increased intra-abdominal pressure, such as in individuals with **chronic obstructive pulmonary disease (COPD)** and liver failure with ascites (build-up of fluid within the abdomen)
- Neurologic causes, such as congenital (from birth) neurologic problems including spina bifida (myelomeningocele) and spinal cord lesions.

56. Do men have to deal with urinary incontinence problems also?

Although much more media attention and literature is spent discussing incontinence as it pertains to females, men also suffer from urinary incontinence but in smaller numbers. This is in contrast to overactive bladder (OAB), where more men than women in their 60s and 70s are affected. In OAB, although the risk increases with age when compared to women, men with OAB tend to remain dry. SUI is uncommon in men, but when it does occur, usually it is related to a surgical intervention, most commonly radical prostatectomy (removal of the entire prostate) and less commonly transurethral prostatectomy (removal of the prostate through the urethra). In both of these procedures, there may be some damage to the **sphincter**

Congenital

existing at birth; refers to physical traits, conditions, diseases, or anomalies, malformations, etc.

Pelvic inflammatory disease (PID)

acute or chronic pus-forming inflammation of female pelvic structures due to infection by *Neisseria ghonorrhea*, *Chlamydia trachomatis*, and other sexually transmitted diseases.

Chronic obstructive pulmonary disease (COPD)

general term used for diseases with permanent or temporary narrowing of small bronchi in the lungs.

Sphincter mechanism

valve that controls urine flow.

mechanism during the surgery that doesn't fully recover, leaving the individual with urinary incontinence. It is not uncommon for men to have SUI the first month or so after a radical prostatectomy. Most men will regain continence by one month after the procedure. In some men, however, it may take longer than a month to regain control and a small percentage of men will have a persistent lack of urinary control.

As with women suffering from urinary incontinence, men with incontinence need to undergo a formal evaluation to determine the type of incontinence and to modify any exacerbating factors. Surgical intervention may also be performed for men suffering from urinary incontinence.

57. What should be done before my physician formally diagnoses me with SUI?

Kathy's comment:

Since I work with urologists, I was able to bypass any primary care workup and go directly to a specialty exam. I was seen by one of the physicians in my practice who has a special interest in urinary incontinence. He took a complete history and physical examination. Emphasis was placed on the pelvic exam to try to assess the adequacy of urethral support. A urinalysis was also performed to make sure I was not infected or inflamed. My urologist believed that my examination to that point suggested that my urine leakage was of the variety that would be considered "genuine stress urinary incontinence." Nevertheless, my urologist explained to me that since we were contemplating a surgical repair, that cystoscopy with urodynamic testing should be done. These were done to measure how well the bladder muscle works and that there were no other unexpected findings. I can safely say that the cystoscopy and urodynamics were easily tolerated from a patient's perspective.

There are several components to the evaluation of urinary incontinence and the identification of the type of incontinence. The evaluation starts with a complete history including: a urologic history, neurologic history, medical and surgical history, and sexual history. The history is often facilitated by having you complete such things as voiding diaries (see Question 27) and quality-of-life questionnaires, so that your doctor may be able to assess the severity and frequency of your symptoms and their impact on your quality of life. A physical examination is important and includes a pelvic and rectal examination, and a sensory and neurologic examination. The pelvic examination is performed to evaluate the health of the vaginal tissues, and to examine for leakage and urethral mobility with a **Valsalva maneuver**. The rectal examination is performed to assess for severe constipation and to check for any rectal masses. A neurologic examination is performed to ensure that the cause of your urinary troubles is not of a neurologic origin. In addition, to determine the degree of leakage your physician may ask you to weigh the pads you wear when you have leaked to gauge the severity of leakage. The laboratory examination consists of a urinalysis and culture to rule out stones, tumors, and infection as the source of your symptoms. Blood tests may also be indicated and may include tests to evaluate your blood sugar and kidney function. Depending on your examination and history, radiologic studies such as a renal/bladder **ultrasound** may be indicated. A renal/bladder ultrasound is a noninvasive test that can evaluate your kidneys and bladder and assess how well you empty your bladder. In select

Valsalva maneuver

any forced expiratory effort ("strain") against a closed airway; used to study cardiovascular effects as well as post-strain responses.

Ultrasound

a noninvasive test using radiowaves to assess bladder emptying capacity.

cases, the physician may wish to perform a cystoscopy (see Question 18). A cystoscopy is warranted in individuals with blood cells in the urine, those with prior incontinence procedures, or those deemed to be at risk for bladder cancer. Urodyamic studies may be needed in more complex cases and in those individuals with a history of prior pelvic surgery (see Question 58).

58. What is a urodynamic study?

Kathy's comment:

When I had my urodynamic study, I started with an empty bladder. A small catheter was placed into my bladder to fully empty it and measure how much urine was left after I had gone to the bathroom. Then my bladder was filled with water and different measurements were taken. After those numbers were obtained, a uroflow study was done. For this test you just sit on a commode seat and empty your bladder. The machine does the rest.

A urodynamic study is a special test that is used to determine how the bladder and urethral muscles work. It evaluates both jobs of the bladder: the storage job and the emptying job. In addition, it can evaluate how well the urethra functions. There are several different parts of a urodynamic study; not all of the different parts are always needed to make a diagnosis.

The urodynamic study may be performed in the office or in a specialized outpatient surgery area. The procedure does not require any special preparation. Your doctor may ask you to arrive for the test with a full bladder.

Uroflow

the urine stream; measured during urodynamic studies.

The test often will start with a simple **uroflow**. The doctor will ask you to urinate into a specialized collecting device that is able to measure how fast you are urinating. After you have urinated, a special catheter is placed inside of the bladder, and the physician will note if any urine is left behind after you urinate. This measurement is called the postvoid residual. The catheter is taped in place. Sometimes the physician may also place a small catheter into the rectum to allow for measuring of pressures within your abdomen. Also, the physician may place some small patches, called **skin patch electrodes**, around the anus. These patches measure the activity in the muscle around the anus. This activity reflects the activity of your pelvic floor muscles, which also surround the urethra, and the study is called **electromyography**. Once all of the catheters and patches are in place and secured, the test will begin. The catheter that goes into your bladder has two channels; one channel is connected to a pressure monitor and the other channel allows for filling of your bladder. Your bladder may be filled with a sterile dye to allow the doctor to intermittently take pictures of your bladder using an x-ray, **fluoroscopy**. Your doctor will select the rate at which he/she chooses to fill your bladder. The doctor will ask you to inform him/her when you first feel the urge to urinate and when you feel a strong urge. That could be defined as when you would pull your car over to the side of the road to urinate if you were driving. The volumes of fluid in your bladder will be noted at each of these times. Periodically during the study, your doctor may ask you to bear down, Valsalva, or give a big cough. During this period he/she will look for leakage of urine, for stress incontinence, and will record the pressures at which the leakage occurred, and if it did occur, the Valsalva leak point pressure. The pressure monitor will also detect any overactive bladder contractions

Skin patch electrodes

a noninvasive, no pain method used in testing muscle activity or pressures involving a flat adhesive patch with embedded wires.

Electromyography

type of noninvasive test using skin patches to measure the activity in the muscles.

Fluoroscopy

a test that visualizes of tissues and deep structures of the body by x-ray.

that may be present, and your doctor may ask you if you feel the need to urinate periodically during the study to see if you sense these overactive bladder contractions and also whether leakage occurs with these contractions. When your bladder feels full and you have a strong urge to urinate, your doctor will have you urinate. If the patch electrodes were placed, the doctor will watch the activity in your pelvic floor muscles on a monitor as you are urinating. Normally when you start to void, the pelvic floor muscles relax and when you are done urinating, they tighten up again. There are several technical terms that reflect the different phases of the study:

Cystometrogram (CMG)

a component of the urodynamic study when your bladder is being filled and the pressures within the bladder are being measured.

Cystometrogram (CMG)—A CMG is the component of the study when your bladder is being filled and the pressures within the bladder are being measured. This part is used to determine if the bladder capacity is normal and whether there are any overactive bladder contractions. When you bear down (Valsalva), the pressure at leakage (the valsalva leak point pressure) is measured, and this measurement is used to help determine the type of stress incontinence that you have. Low Valsalva leak point pressures are indicative of failure of adequate closure of the urethra (see Question 54) whereas a high Valsalva leak point pressure indicates genuine stress urinary incontinence.

Electromyography is the measurement of the activity in the pelvic floor muscles through the use of skin patch electrodes or in some cases needle electrodes placed into the muscle. The electrodes are usually placed around the anus.

Pressure flow study

a specialized study used to assess whether there is any obstruction to the outflow of urine.

Pressure flow study is a specialized study that is used to assess whether or not there is any obstruction to the outflow of urine. This study measures that maximum bladder pressure during voiding and the maximum urine flow rate, and plots these numbers on a graph to determine if obstruction is present.

Videourodynamics is the use of intermittent fluoroscopy (taking x-ray pictures) during the urodynamic study. This is often helpful in assessing the mobility of the urethra and the support to the bladder and in assessing for other abnormalities such as bladder or urethral **diverticula** and vesicoureteral reflux (urine passing backwards from the bladder to the kidneys).

Not all individuals require urodynamic studies prior to treating their bladder and/or incontinence problems, but in some individuals, urodynamics are clearly indicated. Those individuals who are believed to have an overactive bladder and who do not respond to appropriate medical therapy, individuals with bladder and/or urine leakage related to a neurologic problem, and individuals who have undergone prior surgery for urinary incontinence are some of those who would benefit from urodynamic studies.

59. Should every patient undergo urodynamic studies prior to having surgery for urinary incontinence?

There are certain groups of patients who suffer from urinary incontinence who should have urodynamic studies prior to undergoing surgery for urinary incontinence. On the other hand, there is a large group of individuals who can undergo surgery for urinary incontinence safely and surely without a prior urodynamic evaluation. Typically, the individuals who do not need pre-operative urodynamic studies are young

Videourodynamics
use of intermittent fluoroscopy (taking x-ray pictures) during the urodynamic study.

Diverticula
pouch or sac opening from a tubular or saccular organ such as the gut or bladder.

healthy women with a clinical history and physical examination suggestive of stress urinary incontinence. If your urologist or urogynecologist is unclear as to the specific reasons for your urine leakage, then urodynamic studies will prove helpful in determining the cause of your leakage. In addition, if there is a question of mixed urinary incontinence, such as overactive bladder plus stress urinary incontinence, the urodynamic studies will often demonstrate this clearly. In complex patients, such as those with a history of prior surgery for urinary incontinence, a urodynamic study is often very helpful.

NONOPERATIVE TREATMENT OPTIONS

60. My medical doctor says that I am high risk for surgery. If I don't want to jump right into an operative procedure for SUI, are there any medical options that I could try first?

There is currently no single medication or class of medications approved by the FDA for use in stress urinary incontinence. That said, there are a few medications in three different classes that have been used by medical professionals that may have a successful effect on stress urinary incontinence (see Table 5).

The first class of drugs is called **alpha receptor agonists**, or alpha agonists. These medications cause the muscles around the urethra (the sphincter muscles) to tighten (contract). Unfortunately, their action is not limited to the sphincter muscles and they can cause tightening of

Alpha receptor agonists

type of medication that causes the muscles around the urethra, the sphincter muscles, to tighten or contract; may also cause tightening of the muscles that surround arteries and thus result in high blood pressure.

the muscles that surround arteries causing contraction of these and resulting in high blood pressure.

The second class of drugs that are frequently used is estrogens. **Estrogens** may be taken orally or be applied topically (on the skin) to the urethra. Most physicians recommend the use of topical estrogen therapy particularly in light of the recent media attention to the increased risk of breast cancer with the use of oral therapy. With topical therapy, you apply a small dab of the estrogen cream to the distal urethra, by applying it to the outside skin of the vaginal wall. This estrogen works locally to make the urethral tissue healthier. This health of the urethral tissue helps with continence.

Estrogens

a class of drugs, orally or topically applied, used to make the urethral tissue healthier.

The third class of medications that may be used to treat SUI is the **tricyclic antidepressants**. There are two medications in this group that are used for purposes of urinary incontinence, amitriptyline (Elavil) and imipramine (Tofranil). These medications work to lower the bladder pressure by relaxing the bladder muscle and also simultaneously cause tightening of the sphincter muscle.

Tricyclic antidepressants

a class of medications used to lower the bladder pressure by relaxing the bladder muscle and also tighten the sphincter muscle.

Table 5 Types of medications used to treat SUI

Classification	Medication	Pharmacologic Action
Alpha-agonists	Ephedrine Pseuodoephedrine	Increases urethral closure pressure
Estrogens	Estradiol	Thickens urethral lining
Tricyclic antidepressants	Amitriptyline/imipramine	Lowers bladder pressure, and tightens bladder neck

61. *What new medical options are being investigated by the FDA that are specifically for SUI?*

For the first time, there is a medication that is currently under investigation for use in SUI. Called **Duloxetine**, it was developed and is being studied by Lilly Pharmaceuticals. The FDA's initial evaluation of Duloxeline was not favorable. It remains to be seen whether or not Lilly will proceed with further investigation of Doloxetine for stress urinary incontinence. This medication is similar to some antidepressants, but has been found to have an effect on the bladder and urethra. By increasing the amount of a chemical—serotonin—this medication is able to relax the bladder and tighten the bladder outlet, which is the muscle around the urethra. As with many medications, it will also have other uses in medicine, specifically for individuals suffering from depression. The medication will not cause a permanent change and will need to be taken on a regular basis. Preliminary studies have demonstrated that individuals with SUI taking this medication experience about a 50% improvement in the number of stress-related urinary leakage episodes that they experience. In addition, patients believed that they had an improvement in their quality of life. This medication is not without side effects, however. The most distressing side effect of it is nausea, and it can occur in up to 75% of individuals taking the medication. In a large number of people the nausea will resolve, but it may take up to 12 weeks for it to go away.

Duloxetine

a type of medication for stress urinary incontinence that is not yet approved by the FDA. Side effect: nausea.

MINIMALLY INVASIVE OPTIONS

62. A friend of mine really suffered with urinary incontinence, to the point where it was difficult for her to socialize. Now she is dry. She says that her doctor fixed her without the need for surgery and that all she had was an injection in the office. Is this possible?

Injection therapy is a possible treatment for SUI; however, unlike many of the other therapies described in the previous questions in this book, it is useful in only a limited group of individuals. Injection therapy has only proven to be of some benefit to individuals with Type III SUI. It is not effective in those with genuine stress incontinence or urethral hypermobility. Individuals with Type III SUI typically have a history of prior procedures for SUI, prior pelvic surgery, or pelvic radiation. Typically, a urodynamic study is performed to ensure that Type III SUI is present. If you are a candidate for injection therapy, there are two procedures that may be performed: periurethral or transurethral injection. In the **periurethral** approach a needle filled with the agent to be injected is inserted alongside the urethra and the material injected. In the **transurethral** approach, a cystoscope (see Question 18) is inserted into the urethra and a thin, long needle is advanced through the cystoscope and into the urethra. The chemical is then injected into the urethra. The goal of the agent that is injected is to act as a "bulking agent"

Periurethral injection

a type of shot where a needle filled with the agent to be injected is inserted alongside the urethra and the material injected.

Transurethral injection

a type of shot where a cystoscope is inserted into the urethra and a small, long needle is advanced through the cystoscope and into the urethra; the chemical is then injected into the urethra.

Table 6   Agents used to treat urinary incontinence

Agent	FDA Approval	Success Rate/Particle Migration
Autologous fat	Not required	Variable/May migrate, causing fat embolus
Autologous collagen	Not required	Variable/Skin scar at harvest site
GAX collagen (Contigen® Bard®)	Approved 1991	Variable/Absorbed over time/need skin test
Durasphere® (Boston Scientific)	Approved 2000	Variable/No absorption, may migrate

providing compression against the urethra. Such procedures have been utilized since the early 1970s. The success rates with injection therapy are variable and range from very poor to very good. Careful patient selection improves the success rate. More than one injection may be required to improve or cure the urinary incontinence. Depending on the agent used, additional injections may be needed in the future. Over the years there have been four popular bulking agents, which are outlined in Table 6.

Another chemical named Deflux® is under investigation for use in urinary incontinence. It is currently approved for use in the treatment of vesicoureteral reflux.

63. What is the best choice of injectable agent for Type III SUI today?

Currently, the two most common injectable agents used by urologists and urogynecologists are GAX collagen (Contigen® Bard®) and Durasphere® (Boston

Scientific). Other therapies, such as Teflon™, that were popular in Europe have never gained acceptance in the United States. Teflon™ is associated with a significant inflammatory reaction around the particles and the Teflon particles have been shown to migrate to areas such as the brain and lungs. Injectable autologous fat is limited by the need for harvesting of fat cells from the patient and the fact that the fat cells break down over time; therefore, it does not provide for a long-standing cure. Autologous (occurring naturally) collagen also carries the need for harvesting and is limited by the breaking down of autologous collagen over time. Thus, this technique is not durable over the long term either. GAX collagen is collagen derived from a cow. Since cow collagen is not like our own collagen it is not broken down as quickly. Because GAX collagen is not derived from a human body, you must be skin tested prior to using it to make sure that you are not allergic to it. A skin test is performed and if there is no reaction, then you may undergo the collagen injection.

Duraspheres are small carbon beads that are used as bulking agents. Since these are not derived from a human or animal source, there is no need to perform skin testing. These beads do not break down like collagen and fat, so they have the advantage of potential improved durability. These small beads may migrate, however. They have not been identified in the lung, but have been found in the lymph nodes. The implication of this migration is not yet well known.

64. What new minimally-invasive surgical options for stress urinary incontinence are in clinical trials and may soon be released in the United States?

There is a very different therapy for stress urinary incontinence now being evaluated. It is neither a surgical nor medical therapy. This new therapy uses radiofrequency energy to "remold" a poorly functioning and poorly supported bladder and urethra that has lost the ability to snap shut effectively. **Radiofrequency** energy is a form of electromagnetic energy which is almost a generic term for electricity. It is a reproducible and easily controlled form of energy. Radiofrequency energy has been used for remodeling of tissue in other surgical specialties. There are two systems that are currently being tested in clinical trials; one is the SUR*X system and the other the Novasys system. The SUR*X is an operative system that utilizes probes that can be positioned through either a transvaginal or laparoscopic route. The vaginal route seems to be the patient preference as it is less invasive. What the procedure actually does is restructure the support tissues by denaturing proteins, which makes them shorter and stiffer and thus less likely to allow urethral movement during Valsalva maneuvers. The Novasys is an office-based system and does not require anesthesia to perform. The treatment session takes about 20 minutes and the patient is able to sit in a special chair during the procedure. The Novasys is a specialized catheter that is equipped with small curved probes that insert into the soft tissue around the urethra, allowing for the transmission of radiofrequency waves that will remold the poorly supported bladder outlet to make it tight again.

Radiofrequency

a form of electromagnetic energy that is almost a generic term for electricity.

65. What are the treatment options available for men with postprostatectomy urinary incontinence?

It is important to remember that the diagnosis of **postprostatectomy urinary incontinence** cannot really be made until at least 6 to 12 months after the radical prostatectomy. This is an important point, as it is easy for patients to become distraught right after surgery when they experience leakage of urine. Although complete continence in the immediate post-operative period after radical prostatectomy would be wonderful, it is frequently not the case. Lack of continence immediately after surgery does not bode a poor prognosis. During the removal of the prostate there may be weakening of the pelvic floor muscles and it will take time for these muscles to strengthen. Strengthening of these muscles can be accomplished by the use of Kegel exercises (see Questions 29–31). Initially, these exercises may be combined with a medication that tightens the bladder neck muscles as well as medications that relax the bladder. In those individuals with leakage that persists, your urologist will often perform a cystoscopy (see Question 18) to ensure that there is no narrowing at the area where the bladder was sewn to the urethra, bladder neck contracture. Bladder neck contractures may cause difficulty in emptying one's bladder completely and result in overflow incontinence. In the absence of a bladder neck contracture, if urinary incontinence persists then there are several procedures available to help promote dryness.

Postprostatectomy urinary incontinence
leakage of urine in men who have had a prostatectomy; in most cases, this resolves after the pelvic muscles heal.

- Collagen injections: This is often a first-line therapy for males with postprostatectomy urinary incontinence because it is minimally invasive. Collagen is a normal part of our body and is part of our skin and bones. The collagen used for urinary incontinence is not derived from a human; however, it is derived from a cow. The limitations of collagen are that it is broken down by our body over time and that because it is derived from a different animal one may be sensitive or allergic to it. Thus, as the collagen is broken down, incontinence may recur and repeat injections may be necessary. Prior to injection of the collagen, a skin test must be obtained to ensure that one is not allergic to the collagen. The collagen injection is performed through the cystoscope. The cystoscope may be passed through a small hole made in the lower part of your abdomen extending into the bladder (antegrade approach) or through the urethra (retrograde approach). Once the cystoscope is properly positioned, a long, skinny needle is inserted through the scope into the proximal urethra and bladder neck area and the collagen injected until the urethra closes. The procedure takes about 30 minutes and may be performed under **local anesthesia**, a short-acting spinal anesthetic or intravenous sedation. The patient is discharged to home the same day without a catheter. The three limitations of collagen are: (1) the breakdown of collagen limits its long-term durability; (2) approximately 20% of individuals will have troubles voiding after collagen injection; and (3) the injection of collagen may lead to the development of overactive bladder symptoms including urgency, frequency, and nocturia.

Local anesthesia

a short-acting spinal anesthetic or intravenous sedation.

- The male sling: Other questions discuss in great detail the sling procedure for stress urinary incontinence in women (see Questions 74–84). The sling procedure has truly revolutionized surgery for SUI in females. This concept has been applied to men with postprostatectomy urinary incontinence with favorable results. Since the male anatomy is different than the female anatomy, the technique has undergone modifications to make it usable in males. There is actually a specialized kit produced by American Medical Systems that contains a sling derived from pig skin as well as the necessary equipment for the procedure. Male slings typically use bone anchors for securing the sling.

- Artificial urinary sphincter: The sphincter muscle is a muscle that surrounds the urethra just distal (that is, situated away from) to the tip of the prostate. During a radical prostatectomy, as your urologist removes the prostate and the tissue immediately around it, there may be trauma or damage to the pelvic floor muscles and the urethral sphincter. If the muscle(s) are weakened, then the use of pelvic floor muscle exercises may serve to strengthen them. In certain cases, however, the muscles are unable to regain enough strength to prevent urine leakage. If after six months leakage persists, the likelihood of the muscles regaining sufficient strength is low and you may consider other procedures that promote continence. The artificial sphincter is a specialized, three-piece hydraulic device (see Figure 8). It is composed of a cuff, a pump, and a reservoir. The cuff mimics your own natural sphincter muscle. It is placed around the urethra near the level of the bladder neck. The pump is positioned in the scrotum and the reservoir is placed in the abdomen. All of these pieces and the tubing that connects them are

Male (midsagittal section)

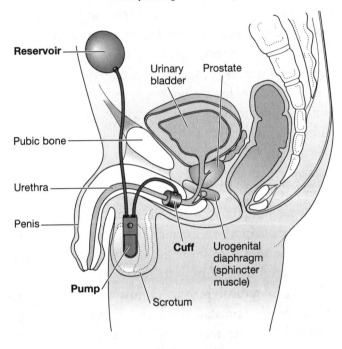

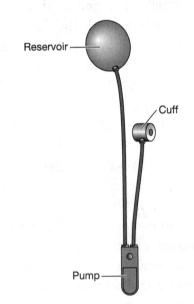

Artificial sphinchter

Figure 8

concealed under the skin. At rest, the cuff is filled with sterile fluid and thus remains in a closed position, as it applies pressure to the urethra. When one feels the urge to urinate, one presses the pump in the scrotum. By pressing the pump, one is actively transferring fluid out of the cuff and into the reservoir. As the cuff deflates, the pressure around the urethra decreases, allowing the urethra to open and urination to occur. The cuff automatically reinflates within a minute or so. The surgical procedure takes about two hours and you are hospitalized for one night. The sphincter is left deactivated for six to eight weeks until all of the healing has occurred. You are then instructed regarding proper use of the sphincter. The success rate of the procedure approaches 90% when defining an end result as total dryness or the use of a mini-pad for protection. There are some risks associated with placement of a sphincter and include: (1) injury to the urethra, (2) malfunction of the device (10%–15%); (3) **erosion** and infection, and (4) new onset of overactive bladder symptoms. Erosion and infection require immediate removal of the sphincter. As with all surgical procedures, it is important that you discuss the risks and benefits in detail with your surgeon.

Erosion
when the pubovaginal sling migrates from its position between the urethra and the vagina and relocates in one of the two organs.

66. What are the surgical options for women with stress urinary incontinence?

There are a variety of surgical options for women suffering from stress urinary incontinence (SUI). The surgical approach to the treatment of SUI has evolved over the last five decades to improve the efficacy and to be less invasive. This evolution reflects the prevalence of this problem in the United States, with an estimated 14 to 18 million American women suffering from SUI at a cost of 10 to 20 billion dollars. Consequently, if surgical procedures provided higher cure rates and were less invasive, the costs related to SUI would be decreased.

The types of surgery for SUI can be broadly defined by how the procedure is performed:

- Purely vaginal—through an incision in the vagina near the proximal urethra and bladder neck.
- Transvaginal needle—via the passage of a needle from the abdominal wall into the vagina or vice versa.
- Open abdominal—through an abdominal incision.
- Laparoscopic—through several tiny abdominal incisions utilitizing a specialized telescope and working instruments.
- Sling procedures—the use of a material passed under the urethra to act as a hammock.
- Injectable agents—the injection of a material either through the urethra or into the tissue outside of the urethra.

This variety of procedures available reflects a continued effort to develop a procedure that is efficacious (beneficial), associated with minimal side effects and risks, and allows the patient to return to full activity quicker (minimally invasive), as well as the fact that there are different types of SUI, which may require different forms of treatment.

In answer to a questionnaire asking what brought her to the decision to go ahead and undergo surgical correction for her stress incontinence, one patient commented:

The symptoms had increased to the point where I was leaking on a daily basis. I was wearing a pad every day.

The turning point was one weekend when I was sitting in the car (vinyl seats, thank God) and all of a sudden I was leaking without any warning. I wet myself in the car and the worst part was I couldn't stop it. That lack of control made me very anxious and it was then that I decided that I needed to get control of my life back and it was time to seek help.

Another patient who was asked, "What were your expectations of surgery before you had it?" replied as follows:

I met with my surgeon to discuss the surgery after he had evaluated me. He was very optimistic about the success of the surgery for me. I must admit that I was hoping to be completely dry, but I had my doubts. Could someone who leaked as much as me become totally dry? It sounded too good to be true. My doctor clearly explained the procedure to me and allowed me to ask questions regarding the surgery and the post-operative course so I felt that I was pretty well prepared. I am a pretty organized person so I had made my list of questions regarding the surgery and my doctor was willing to go through them with me. This made things easier for me.

67. What is the Kelly procedure for SUI?

The **Kelly procedure** is one of the most common procedures performed by gynecologists who treat SUI. Today, it is usually performed in conjunction with a vaginal or "partial" hysterectomy in patients who have a combination of uterine descent and urinary leakage. This procedure has been used since the early 1900s. One of the most attractive aspects of this procedure is that it may be performed completely through the vagina. There is no need for any abdominal incisions. The operation consists of a small incision in the vagina. The incision is placed where the bladder neck

Kelly procedure
a surgical procedure usually performed in conjunction with a vaginal or "partial" hysterectomy in patients who have a combination of uterine descent and urinary leakage.

and urethra are located anterior (i.e., at the surface of the body) to the vagina. After the incision is made, the underlying tissue is freed from the vaginal wall exposing the weakened pelvic muscles. These muscles are then sewn together to create a "buttress" that supports the bladder and urethra to help prevent urine leakage. The vaginal incision is then closed. A vaginal pack may be left in place overnight, depending on your surgeon's preference.

68. Who is a candidate for the Kelly procedure and what are the risks?

The best candidates for the Kelly procedure are women who:

- Have finished having children.
- Have not reached menopause, as the tissue tends to be healthier in premenopausal women.
- Have genuine stress urinary incontinence.

If these three criteria are met, the procedure will have the highest success rate. Since the Kelly procedure is purely a vaginal procedure when performed as the sole-procedure, it is considered to be a low-risk procedure.

The Kelly procedure has a very low complication rate, as serious complications occur in less than 1%. The risk of developing an overactive bladder (see Question 7) is less than 6%. Compared to some other procedures, there is less blood loss and the risk of long-term voiding troubles is almost nonexistent. Nevertheless, it is a surgical procedure and thus there are the risks that accompany all surgical procedures, including bleeding and infection.

Bleeding: Since the Kelly procedure involves incision of and dissection around the vagina, there is the risk of bleeding from the vagina and the surrounding tissue. When this occurs, it is often treated successfully by placement of a vaginal pack to provide compression. The pack is typically removed the following day. If bleeding persists despite packing, then the area is examined under anesthesia and the site of bleeding identified if possible and the bleeding controlled. Rarely, the site of bleeding will not be identified and an angiography will be needed to identify the source of bleeding and to **embolize** it. Angiography is a radiologic procedure whereby a needle is placed into an artery and a small open tubing, an **angiocatheter**, is passed into the artery until it is at the desired location. Then dye is injected into the tubing to allow for visualization of other surrounding arteries. If there is a bleeding artery, the angiocatheter can be moved until it is just before the bleeding artery and a specialized device, a coil, can be passed through the angiocatheter into a position within the artery just before the site of bleeding. The coil serves to obstruct the artery to prevent further bleeding. A vaginal **hematoma** may occur if there is significant bleeding. This is a collection of blood underneath the vaginal incision. Hematomas resolve with time, but may lead to increased postoperative discomfort, prolonged bloody vaginal drainage, and, rarely, may become infected.

Infection: A vaginal **abscess** is a collection of pus under the vaginal tissue. Treatment of an abscess

Embolism

obstruction or occlusion of a vessel.

Angiocatheter

a small tube is inserted into a blood vessel and dye is injected into it, so that the surrounding blood vessels and capillaries can be visualized to determine if there is a leak.

Hematoma

a collection of blood that forms in a tissue, organ, or body space as a result of a broken blood vessel.

Abscess

collection of pus under the skin.

requires opening of the incision in the vagina, drainage of the pus, and packing of the space to allow the tissue to heal and to prevent the pus from reaccumulating. Urinary tract infections may occur related to instrumentation, such as a cystoscopy and/or an indwelling **catheter**. These are treated with the appropriate antibiotics.

Urinary Retention: Urinary retention, the inability to urinate on one's own, may occur with any procedure for SUI. In most cases, it is transient and will resolve. Rarely will it persist and require a revision of the surgical procedure. For those women who are unable to urinate after surgery, they are taught clean intermittent catheterization (see Question 50), which they perform until they are voiding spontaneously on their own. Sometimes, if you cannot urinate on your own right after the surgery, your doctor will send you home with a catheter in place for a week, and then have you return to remove the catheter and try to void on your own again. The risk of urinary retention with the Kelly procedure is much less than other surgical procedures for SUI.

69. What is the success rate for the Kelly procedure for SUI?

It is important to remember that the Kelly procedure remains popular today for three reasons. First, it can be performed completely through the vagina, thus avoiding any incisions on the abdomen. The morbidity of a vaginal procedure is much less than that of an abdominal procedure. Second, the Kelly procedure is easy to perform at the same time as a vaginal (partial) hysterectomy. Third,

Catheter

a tubular instrument especially designed to be passed through the urethra into the bladder to drain the bladder.

it may correct SUI without "burning any bridges." That is, if the procedure fails, it is easy to go back and perform another surgery for the SUI. Although the procedure has an initial cure rate ranging from 31% to 100%, at five years after surgery the success rate drops to 37%.

70. My mother had a transvaginal needle suspension procedure to correct her SUI with good results, but my doctor says that these are not routinely performed anymore. How can that be?

Transvaginal needle suspension procedures were developed in the late 1950s and were very popular in the 1970s and 1980s because they offered a less invasive approach to treating urinary incontinence. There were four major types of **transvaginal needle suspension procedures** that were used to correct SUI: the Pereyra procedure, the Stamey procedure, the Raz procedure, and the Gittes procedure. The Pereyra procedure was the first procedure developed and the remainder continued to modify that surgical technique. The Gittes procedure was the first procedure that did not involve a vaginal incision. The goal of all of these procedures is to provide support to the bladder neck and urethra. Although these procedures were noted to have excellent success rates initially, with cure rates as high as 83%, over the long term the success rates appeared to decrease significantly. Another reason for the lack of persistent enthusiasm for these procedures was the increased understanding of the different types of SUI and the realization that these procedures were ineffective for Type III SUI. Thus, the focus turned to identi-

Transvaginal needle suspension procedures

a type of surgical procedure used to correct SUI in the 1950s–1980s.

Open abdominal procedures for SUI

surgical procedures used to repair a dysfunctional bladder; typically referred to as "retropubic bladder neck suspensions" or more commonly, bladder suspensions.

Marshall Marchetti and Krantz (MMK) procedure

a type of surgical procedure where sutures are placed in the tissue surrounding the urethra and tacked behind the pubic bone, hence the term retropubic; the sutures are placed to provide support to the bladder and bladder neck/proximal urethra so that increases in abdominal pressure will be transmitted to both the bladder and the proximal urethra.

Burch procedure

type of surgery similar to the Marshall Marchetti and Krantz procedure, except that the pubic bone is not used to support the bladder and bladder neck; rather the sutures are placed in some strong tissue a little more lateral, in the Cooper's ligament.

fying a procedure that was durable and could also treat Type III SUI.

71. What are the open abdominal procedures for correction of SUI?

Open abdominal procedures for the correction of SUI, like the Kelly procedure, have stood the test of time. They are still in use today, but are usually performed in conjunction with another abdominal or pelvic procedure such as a "total" hysterectomy by a gynecologist. These open procedures for SUI are typically referred to as "retropubic bladder neck suspensions" or more commonly, bladder suspensions. These procedures have been used since the late 1940s. Currently, there are two bladder suspensions that are commonly used, the **Marshall Marchetti and Krantz (MMK) procedure** and the Burch procedure. Both procedures are typically performed through a c-section (Pfannenstiel) incision. The incision is located about one inch above the pubic bone and is made transversely in a normal skin crease. Postoperatively, the incision is often covered by regrowth of pubic hair or is hidden in a normal skin crease. Although these procedures are referred to as abdominal procedures, the abdominal cavity is not opened, rather, these procedures are performed in the pelvis. Once the pelvis is entered, the bladder and urethra are identified. For the MMK procedure, sutures are placed in the tissue surrounding the urethra and tacked behind the pubic bone, hence the term "retropubic." The sutures are placed to provide support to the bladder and bladder neck/proximal urethra so that increases in abdominal pressure will be transmitted to both the bladder and the proximal urethra. The open **Burch procedure** is performed in a similar manner, except that the pubic bone is not used to support the bladder and bladder neck, rather the sutures are placed in some strong tissue a little more lateral, Cooper's ligament.

72. Who are candidates and what are the risks of these open bladder suspensions?

The best candidates for these open bladder suspensions are women who fulfill three requirements:

- They are finished having children.
- They suffer from genuine SUI.
- There is no element of Type III SUI (see Question 51).

Although not a strict contraindication to treatment, women with mixed urinary incontinence, SUI plus urge incontinence (see Question 53), also have a lower continence rate with open bladder suspensions compared to those with pure stress incontinence. In 60% to 70% of women with mixed urinary incontinence, the OAB symptoms will resolve after surgery, but 30% will continue to have OAB symptoms. Thus, those women with mixed urinary incontinence should have their OAB symptoms adequately treated prior to considering SUI surgery.

Those individuals who are at increased risk for failure of a Burch or MMK include postmenopausal females, those who have undergone a prior hysterectomy, and those who have undergone prior anti-incontinence surgery. Those individuals with Type III SUI have a hyper chance of failure with the Burch or MMK.

Although the risk of serious complications with these procedures is low (less than 5%), it is important that you are aware of some of the risks and how they are managed if they do occur. The most common complications after the MMK and Burch are wound complications (infection, hematoma, hernia, and wound separation) and urinary tract infections. Injury to the urinary tract, the bladder, urethra and/or ureter is rare, although a more serious complication.

Injury to the bladder or urethra: This risk is low, approximately 3%. Bladder injuries include tears in the bladder (0.7%), and sutures placed through the bladder or urethra may also catch the Foley catheter in 0.3%. Often a bladder injury will heal on its own and will only require that the drainage tube(s), Foley catheter, and/or suprapubic tube be left in place until the bladder is healed. If a suture is placed through the bladder and it is not recognized at the time of surgery, it may cause stones to form in the bladder and this may lead to recurrent urinary tract infections, blood in the urine, and discomfort with frequency of voiding. Ureteral injuries can be a bit more serious but are less frequent. Ureteral obstruction occurs in 0.1% of patients. Although this is rare, it may occur more commonly with the Burch procedure and can be treated with removal of the stitches and placement of a ureteral stent. The ureteral stent is removed at a later time when the swelling has resolved.

Fistula

a communication between two organs; for example, a vesicovaginal fistula, whereby the bladder and vagina are connected by a small, open tract that allows urine to pass from the bladder into the vagina.

Fistula formation: Fistula formation is rare, and is less in 0.3% of patients undergoing an MMK and less frequent in those undergoing a Burch procedure. A **fistula** is a communication between two organs, such as a vesicovaginal fistula, whereby the bladder and vagina are connected by a small, open tract that allows urine to pass from the bladder into the vagina.

Infections can be simple or complicated. Skin infections are treated with antibiotics. If there is a collection of pus under the incision (which is an abscess), the incision needs to be opened, the abscess drained, and the wound packed to prevent the abscess from returning. Rarely, the abscess may form deeper in the pelvis, and this is often treated with the placement of a small drain into the abscess to drain the pus. More often the infection that occurs is a urinary tract infection. Urinary tract infections occur in 10% to 15% of individuals undergoing these procedures and are treated with antibiotics.

Deep venous thrombosis (DVT): The most common location of a DVT is in your legs. Typically, a DVT presents with lower leg swelling and discomfort in your calf. A DVT is a blood clot in the veins. This is a potentially serious problem because if the blood clot becomes dislodged, it can travel to your lungs and cause a pulmonary embolus (obstruction), which can be lethal. Thus, your surgeon will often either give you an injection of a blood thinner or put specialized stockings and inflatable devices on your lower legs while you are in the hospital to prevent a DVT. If you develop a DVT, you will need to be put on blood thinners for a period of time to dissolve the clot.

Urinary retention: Urinary retention is the inability to spontaneously pass urine on your own. This problem is seen immediately after the surgery and occurs in about 20% of individuals undergoing an MMK or Burch procedure. It is often transient and resolves within a month after the surgery. Individuals with normal bladder function prior to surgery will be able to void on their own without difficulty in most cases. Individuals with bladders that do not contract well are at greater risk for voiding troubles after surgery.

Overactive bladder: Overactive bladder, a term used to describe the symptoms of urgency with or without urge incontinence, and often associated with frequency and nocturia occurs in 7% to 27% of individuals undergoing bladder suspensions. Some individuals may have an overactive bladder prior to surgery. It is important to identify this prior to surgery and to treat the overactive bladder to prevent the surgery from worsening the symptoms. If the overactive bladder symptoms occur after surgery, it is important to rule out obstruction to the outflow of urine as a cause. If there is no obstruction, then the overactive bladder symptoms may be treated with medication. If there is an obstruction to the outflow of urine, then surgery is indicated to relieve the obstruction.

MMK-related risks: In addition to the above-mentioned risks the MMK procedure has two unique risks related to the placement of sutures into the pubic bone. One is **osteomyelitis**, which is an infection of the bone. This requires a long course of antibiotics to treat. The other is **osteitis pubis**. Osteitis pubis occurs in about 2.5% of individuals undergoing the MMK procedure. The cause of the condition is not clear. It typically presents 2 to 12 weeks after surgery. Individuals suffering from osteitis pubis present with pain above the pubic bone that may radiate to the thighs and which is made worse by walking or spreading one's legs. Often there is tenderness to touch over the pubic bone. The symptoms may last for a few weeks to several

Osteomyelitis

inflammation of the bone marrow and adjacent bone.

Osteitis pubis

pain above the pubic bone that may radiate to the thighs and is made worse by walking or spreading the legs. There is often tenderness to touch over the pubic bone.

months. Treatment for osteitis pubis starts with bed rest, and includes physical therapy and anti-inflammatory medications, and sometimes steroids. Rarely, a portion of the pubic bone will need to be removed.

73. What is the postoperative course like for the open abdominal procedures?

Postoperatively (after the surgery), patients can be expected to be sore around the incision for a couple of weeks. As time passes, the discomfort will decrease. Your physician will ask that you avoid any strenuous activity and heavy lifting for about a month after the procedure, until the incision has healed completely. A catheter will be placed into the urethra and will remain in place for several days. The Foley catheter is used to drain the bladder until you are moving around and then it is removed. Some physicians will also place a tube directly into the bladder at the time of surgery, called a **suprapubic tube**. This tube exits through the skin on your lower abdomen and has the same purpose as the Foley catheter, but tends to be less irritating. The Foley catheter is removed a day or two after your surgery and a voiding trial (attempt at having you void on your own) is performed. If you are able to void on your own then you are discharged to home. If you are unable to urinate on your own then you are taught how to perform clean intermittent catheterization (CIC; see Question 50), which you perform until you are voiding or your voiding problem is surgically corrected. The advantage of the suprapubic tube is that you can clamp the tube and then unclamp it after you urinate to check to see if you are emptying your bladder completely.

Suprapubic tube

a type of tube placed directly into the bladder at the time of surgery, that exits through the skin on your lower abdomen to drain the bladder; less irritating than a Foley catheter.

74. What are the results a patient can expect after undergoing an open retropubic bladder suspension?

It is important to remember that the MMK and Burch procedures remain popular today for three reasons. First, they can be performed in conjunction with a popular gynecologic procedure, total abdominal hysterectomy (TAH). Second, the procedures are associated with a low risk for complications. Third, and probably most important, is the fact that the procedures are very successful in treating SUI. Therefore, it is very reasonable for a patient to consider having one of these open bladder suspensions at the same time as an abdominal hysterectomy, since it does not add a significant time or risk to the hysterectomy procedure.

The cure rates with the MMK are in the 80% to 86% range, with an additional 3% of individuals having improvement in wetting episodes. Over a 10- to 20-year period about 20% of those who were initially cured will develop recurrent urinary incontinence. The MMK appears to have a better success rate when performed in patients who have not had any prior incontinence surgery.

For the Burch procedure the initial success rates ranging from 71% to 100% have been reported. Continence rates three to seven years after surgery are reported to range from 63% to 89%.

75. Can the Burch procedure be performed in a minimally invasive fashion?

During the last decade or so, great efforts have been made toward the development of less invasive surgical procedures. **Laparoscopy** is the ability to view the

Laparoscopy

a minimally invasive surgical procedure that allows a view of the entire contents of the abdomen through the use of a specialized instrument, which is attached to a light source, camera, and surgical tools that are passed through a small incision under the umbilicus (belly button).

entire contents of the abdomen through the use of a specialized instrument that is attached to a light source, camera, and tiny surgical tools that are passed through a small incision under the umbilicus (belly button). It has allowed for many less invasive procedures to be performed. Through the use of specialized instruments passed through several small incisions in the abdomen, surgeons can perform a variety of procedures without the need for a large abdominal incision. The first laparoscopic Burch procedure was performed in 1991. The laparoscopic approach differs from the traditional open procedure in the type and number of sutures placed. With the laparoscopic approach, two sutures instead of three are placed on each side of the bladder neck and in an effort to decrease operative time; some surgeons are using staples instead of sutures. The laparoscopic procedure appears to also achieve satisfactory continence rates.

When asked, "Did the surgery meet your expectations?" one patient commented:

I was a bit dubious about becoming completely dry with surgery, so when I went through the surgery and found myself completely dry I was ecstatic. The surgery surpassed my expectations. I was totally thrilled with the outcome and would recommend it to anyone who is experiencing problems with incontinence. The benefit of being dry far surpassed the nuisances of the surgery and the recovery period.

Another patient, asked what the recovery period was like, replied:

I had a laparoscopic Burch procedure and the recovery period was pretty uneventful. My doctor had discussed with me prior to surgery that when I woke up from the procedure that I would have both a Foley catheter and a suprapubic tube. I found the Foley catheter to be uncomfortable, but that was removed about five hours after my surgery. The suprapubic tube was left in place for only about four to five days and that was bearable. I was very happy that after the surgery I was able to void on my own, and that the suprapubic tube was removed quickly and that I did not have to perform clean intermittent catheterization. My doctor had warned that there was a small chance that I would have to perform clean intermittent catheterization, so I was prepared for it, but needless to say was very excited that I didn't actually have to do it. With respect to the recovery period I was back to work in 2.5 weeks, but had to refrain from lifting heavy objects for four to six weeks. Since I had the procedure performed laparoscopically, I had only small incisions that did not cause me much discomfort. The only other nuisance that I can recall regarding the procedure was just the hoarseness in my throat when I woke up from surgery. That was related to the breathing tube that was placed and went away in two days.

76. Who are candidates and what are the risks of the laparoscopic Burch procedure?

Kathy's comment:

Knowing the number of surgical procedures available and after discussion with my surgeon, I chose the laparoscopic Burch. He was very comfortable with the procedure and felt that this would be the best option for me. I also agreed with him on these issues. I had no problems with the gas that was used to distend my belly. The only issue I had with postoperative problems was pain in my lower right groin area. I had intermittent pain/discomfort in this area.

Upon investigation by my surgeon, there were no problems discovered and he said to wait one year. He said that small women he had found many times have this discomfort but it usually resolves in about a year. The discomfort was not unbearable and did dissipate in one year.

The best candidates for the laparoscopic Burch are women who fulfill those requirements discussed for an open Burch procedure (see Questions 71–73). Unlike the open Burch procedure, the laparoscopic Burch is used when typically no other intra-abdominal procedures are being performed. The complications related to the laparoscopic Burch are the same as with the open Burch procedure (see Questions 71–73). In addition, there are complications that may occur related to the laparoscopy. Laparoscopy-related complications include injury to intra-abdominal structures such as the intestines, liver, spleen, and blood vessels during placement of the ports. These complications occur in less than 5% of the patients; however, they do require immediate attention to prevent significant blood loss, infection, and further damage.

Subcutaneous emphysema (presence of gas or air under the skin) may occur. The gas that is used to distend the abdomen may track under the skin and result in skin that looks swollen, yet when the skin is pressed the gas can be felt underneath. This problem will resolve with time.

Shoulder pain may occur related to overdistention (filling beyond normal capacity) of the abdominal cavity with gas.

The need to convert the laparoscopic procedure to an open procedure occasionally occurs related to technical difficulties or significant bleeding encountered during the procedure.

77. What is the pubovaginal sling surgery for stress urinary incontinence in women?

Pubovaginal sling

type of surgical procedure that uses the muscles in the pelvis to create a hammock to support the bladder.

Type III stress incontinence

a circumstance where the urethra itself doesn't close, so any increase in bladder pressure overpowers the urethra and causes leakage of urine.

The modern day **pubovaginal sling** is a procedure that was developed by Dr. Edward McGuire. Dr. McGuire and colleagues identified that there were different types of stress urinary incontinence. One that was related to hypermobility of the urethra responded to the open bladder suspension and transvaginal procedures. Another type, the instrinsic sphincter deficiency, **Type III SUI**, did not respond to the traditional procedures. Dr. McGuire embarked upon the development of a procedure that would treat Type III SUI specifically. Historically, the pubovaginal sling as described by Dr. McGuire used a piece of fascia, a strong tissue that overlies muscles, from the abdominal wall, which was placed underneath the urethra to act as a hammock. The fascia had sutures placed on each end, which were passed from the vaginal incision through the pelvis and tied over the abdominal muscles and fascia. These sutures secured the hammock of fascia in place. Care was taken not to tie the sutures too tight. Since this original description there have been a variety of modifications including the use of fascia from other sites on the body and use of synthetic materials has been described. Its initial use was limited to patients that had failed prior incontinence surgery and who had Type III incontinence, but may also be used in those who have classic SUI and also Type III SUI.

78. Who are the most appropriate patients for sling surgery?

There are three major groups of patients who are candidates for sling surgery. The first is the group of women with classic stress urinary incontinence, who leak urine when they cough, laugh, or sneeze, and who are noted to have hypermobility to their urethra. These women also are candidates for the laparoscopic Burch procedure. The second group of patients comprise those with Type III SUI and is a smaller group. This group has typically had prior pelvic or urethral surgery, and are the ones for whom the procedure was specifically designed. The third group is the smallest and accounts for those individuals with neurologic problems related to spinal cord abnormalities. The most common spinal cord abnormality is spina bifida or myelodysplasia. In all of these groups, the women should be finished with childbearing, and if there is an underlying problem with an overactive bladder it is treated prior to the sling procedure.

79. What are the risks and complications associated with pubovaginal sling surgery?

Kathy's comment:

I did not have this surgery, but in my practice it is very widely used. I have seen many patients who have had this procedure done. Although the postoperative complication rate is very low, the most common problem that I have seen is urinary retention. When these patients come back, it is common to have them catheterize themselves for a short period of time. The patient would then fall into my lap, because one of my responsibilities is to teach CIC (clean intermittent catheterization). Some of these patients are distressed because they have just had their indwelling catheter removed and, although not painful, it can be uncomfortable. Not surprisingly, a certain percentage of these patients are very tentative learning CIC. During the teaching process, the patients will frequently confide in me. I can say that many are worried because they feel like the problem may not resolve or worse they may need additional surgery to correct the problem. Fortunately, this is usually not the case.

Overall, the risks of the pubovaginal sling surgery are low. As with all surgical procedures, there is the risk of bleeding, infection, and discomfort. The most important complications of sling procedures are: (1) bladder or urethral injury, (2) urethral obstruction, and (3) symptomatic overactive bladder.

Injury to the bladder and/or urethra is uncommon during a sling procedure. In most cases, when such an injury occurs it is a tear and may be treated conservatively. If the tear is large, the surgeon may elect to leave a Foley catheter in place for a week longer or place a special tube from the abdomen into the bladder, called a suprapubic tube, until the tear has healed.

Symptomatic overactive bladder, manifested as urinary urgency and frequency occurs in 5% to 10% of patients after surgery. This problem is often a short-term problem and is relieved with the use of bladder relaxant medications, called **antimuscarinic agents** (see Question 23), until the symptoms have resolved. Individuals with persistent overactive bladder symptoms should be evaluated for possible urethral obstruction.

Urinary retention (the inability to void on one's own) occurs in less than 3% of individuals after a sling pro-

Antimuscarinic agents

a medication that blocks the effects of the neurotransmitter acetylcholine's action on muscarinic receptors. Muscarinic receptors in the bladder are involved in the control of bladder muscle contraction.

cedure. In most patients this is a short-term problem and resolves within a month after surgery. If you experience urinary troubles immediately after surgery, your surgeon may elect to send you home with an indwelling Foley catheter for an additional week and then remove it in the clinic and see if you can void at that time. If you are unable to void at that time or if your surgeon desires to do so initially, he/she may start you on clean intermittent catheterization (see Question 50). You would continue on the clean intermittent catheterization until you are able to void on your own or until further evaluation and possible surgical correction is indicated. It is believed that you should be voiding spontaneously by eight weeks after a sling surgery, and failure to do so by eight weeks is suggestive of obstruction.

Urethral obstruction is a recognized risk of a sling procedure and occurs in about 5% of individuals. This typically causes problems urinating and urinary retention. Typically, if voiding problems persist after surgery the surgeon will perform a cystoscopy to rule out the possibility of urethral erosion and a urodynamic study to determine if obstruction is present. In the cases of erosion and obstruction, an additional surgical procedure is required. In the setting of erosion, the sling is removed. With obstruction, often the surgical procedure consists of cutting the sling. Often, after this you will be able to void on your own and remain dry.

Erosion of the sling material into the urethra is rare with the use of the rectus fascia, because this fascia is obtained from the abdomen. Erosion is when the sling migrates from its position between the urethra and the vagina into one of these two structures. Although rare, erosion occurs more commonly with synthetic (man-made) slings. If the sling erodes into the urethra it may cause obstruction, discomfort with voiding, or blood in the urine. If your surgeon performs a **cystoscopy**, the sling can be visualized protruding into the urethra. If the sling erodes into the vagina, an infection may develop or there may be bloody drainage from the vagina. A speculum examination will demonstrate the sling protruding into the vaginal cavity. When synthetic material is used for the sling, the risk of erosion and fistula formation is 20%. If an erosion occurs, the sling must be removed.

Cystoscopy

a procedure in which the bladder and urethra are examined through a narrow telescope-like device that is passed through the urethra into the bladder.

Pain with movement can occur in 2% to 3% of patients after sling surgery and is usually on one side or the other, but not on both sides. This pain generally passes in two to three weeks. If the pain is persistent, additional measures such as the injection of a local anesthetic into the area combined with nonsteroidal anti-inflammatories (NSAIDs) such as ibuprofen may be used. If satisfactory relief of the pain does not occur by 10 weeks after surgery, your surgeon may elect to remove the suture knot on the side of your pain.

Other complications include the risk of blood clots developing in your legs (DVT), a wound infection, or a hernia.

80. Why was the classic pubovaginal sling procedure reserved for end–stage patients who had failed other previous therapy?

At the time that the sling was first developed, doctors believed that the transvaginal procedures for SUI were working well for those individuals with genuine stress incontinence. What was needed was a procedure for those individuals with type III SUI and those who had failed a transvaginal procedure. The pubovaginal sling was viewed as a more invasive procedure than the transvaginal procedures and thus its use in individuals with genuine stress incontinence was not adopted early on. Modifications of the procedure to decrease the side effects (morbidity) of the procedure, but not the efficacy, and a generalized comfort with the procedure have led to its greater use. Such modifications include the use of alternative materials for the "hammock," thus avoiding the need for a large abdominal incision, and a greater understanding of the need to keep the hammock loose to prevent obstruction.

81. How is the pubovaginal sling procedure performed?

If a patient meets the criteria for a classic pubovaginal sling, then standard preoperative preparations are started. Typically, a history and physical examination is performed, and depending on the patient's age and overall health status additional tests such as blood tests, a chest x-ray, and an electrocardiogram may be necessary. The final preoperative steps should include an in-depth question and answer period with the surgeon to review all of the potential surgical outcomes. Once this has been performed, a consent for surgery will be obtained. Typically, the patient will be asked to refrain from eating or drinking from midnight on the evening prior to surgery, but will be allowed to take sips of water with any medications if taken routinely.

The surgery is often performed under either a general or spinal/epidural anesthetic. The patient, surgeon, and the anesthesiologist will decide together what type of anesthesia is most appropriate.

Once anesthetized, the patient will be positioned on the bed to facilitate the two components of the surgery: the harvesting of the fascial sling and the placement of the sling. The patient is usually placed in a lithotomy position, whereby the patient's legs are placed into special stirrups, which spread and support the patient's legs. For the rectus fascial sling, a transverse incision (across the width of the body) is made on the lower abdomen and the fascial strip is marked out and then removed. The fascia is sewn back together. A vaginal incision is made to allow for exposure of the bladder neck/proximal urethra. The fascial strip is then positioned under the bladder neck and proximal urethra, and small trocars are placed on each side from the abdominal incision down through the pelvic into the vaginal incision. **Trocars** are tubular instruments that withdraw fluids from the abdomen. The sutures are then grasped in the trocars and retracted (pulled back) up into the abdominal incision. A cystoscopy is then performed to make sure that the sutures are not passing through the bladder (see Question 18). The sutures from each side are then tied together in the midline. Care is taken to position the piece of fascia in the correct position and to avoid tying the stitches too tight. The vaginal and abdominal incisions are then closed. A catheter is placed in the bladder and some packing gauze into the vagina. Typically, the packing material is removed the next morning and the catheter is removed to see if the patient can urinate on their own. Some surgeons will send patients home with the catheter in place for a few days and then ask them to return to clinic to remove the catheter. If the patient is unable to void after the catheter is removed, he or she will be taught CIC (see Question 50), which the patient will continue until he or she is voiding well on their own or the sling is cut.

Trocar

tubular instrument that withdraw fluids from the abdomen during surgery.

82. What is the in-situ vaginal wall sling?

This was one of the first modifications of the sling. This in situ (Latin for "in position") procedure was developed by Dr. Shlomo Raz in the mid 1980s. Dr. Raz was also responsible for refining the transvaginal needle suspension. Instead of using the rectus fascia, Dr. Raz used a segment of the patient's own vaginal wall to act as the hammock. This meant that the sling could be harvested from the same incision in the vagina that would be used for the vaginal component of the repair. The vagina is a very flexible and expandable (called distensible) organ, and the removal of a small segment did not compromise its ability to distend. This modification was associated with a significant decrease in the risk of complications for the patient.

In-situ vaginal wall sling

type of incontinence bladder surgery that uses a segment of the patient's own vaginal wall to act as the hammock to support the bladder.

During the in situ procedure, sutures are placed on the lateral (on the side) edges of the isolated segment of vaginal wall, and they are brought through the pelvis and attached to the anterior abdominal wall. This procedure is actually a combination of the transvaginal needle suspension procedure and the sling procedure. It has been used in both individuals suffering from genuine stress urinary incontinence and Type III stress incontinence.

83. Can't the sling be constructed out of a natural material that is not taken out of my own body?

Once the pubovaginal sling had been demonstrated to be safe, effective, and durable, the next step was to develop ways to improve on the established procedure. One of the limiting factors with the pubovaginal sling

Fascia

a sheet of connective tissue covering or binding together body structures.

is the need to harvest the **fascia**. The fascia was originally taken from the abdominal wall, which meant that a relatively large (by today's standards) incision was needed and this lengthened the recuperation time to heal the wound. The ideal procedure would involve tissue or material that didn't require an incision and that would be strong and durable. A variety of fascial tissues have been tried. The three most common tissues that have been used for the sling include: blood bank cadaveric fascia (tissue from a deceased human), which is stored in the hospital's blood bank; a Tutoplast® treated fascia known as SUSPEND (manufactured by Mentor or Pelvicol™), which is a tissue derived from a pig and prepared by the Bard urologic division. Since these are all nonsynthetic tissues, the risk of erosion is low and they have been shown to be strong.

The advantage of blood bank fascia is that it is stored within the hospital and thus is readily available. However, there are some disadvantages to the use of blood bank cadaveric fascia. These include a very high cost, which is naturally associated with its limited supply. In addition, there is no routine harvesting process and occasionally pieces can be thin and flimsy, and tear apart easily. Finally, and perhaps most concerning, is there is no formal preparation process to remove possible viruses, bacteria, and antigens, which leaves the patient vulnerable to potential inflammatory and infectious processes.

SUSPEND is also cadaveric fascia. However, Mentor has addressed two of the problems that are noted with blood bank fascia. First, the fascia is harvested in a standard manner that produces consistent, thick, strong fascia. Second, the fascia undergoes a cleansing process that ensures that the tissue is safe to use. This specialized process inactivates viruses and other materials that may make the fascia harmful to the patient. Thus, this product has the advantages of cadaveric fascia without the risks.

Xenografts are biologic tissues that are removed from other species. Pelvicol® is such a xenograft. It is pigskin which is strong and durable. In the development of Pelvicol® for use in humans, Bard pretreats the tissue so that the patient won't react to it and there is no risk of infection. This is a strong, durable alternative to human fascia; however, for patients with some religions, this may not be a suitable option.

Xenografts
biologic tissues that are removed from other species and used in human transplantation.

84. Are there any synthetic materials that can be used as material for a sling?

As one would expect the evolution of sling materials has continued to progress. Some choices of synthetic materials that can be used as a sling include: GoreTex®, Mersile, and generic Prolene mesh. Unfortunately, these materials are associated with a higher risk of complications such as erosion and fistula formation. Furthermore, if their removal is required it is much more challenging than the removal of rectus fascia. Thus, there is a tempered enthusiasm for the use of such materials in sling procedures.

Protogen, a synthetic sling, which was used with the "vesica kit," has been taken off of the market. This vesica kit was composed of two relatively new techniques: One was the use of a synthetic material for the sling and the other was the use of bone anchors to avoid the need for an abdominal incision. The bone anchors are like screws that are placed into the pubic bone and the suture of the sling is tied to the bone anchors to secure it rather than to the abdominal wall. Although the initial results with this procedure were favorable, the five-year results did not look as favorable and there were increasing numbers of complications. The most common complication was the erosion of the synthetic material through the urethra and the bladder walls, creating an abnormal communication (called a fistula) that would cause complete uncontrollable loss of urine, which is socially unacceptable. The second group of major complications had to do with bone anchors. Inflammation and infection of the pelvic bones was not uncommon. As you might imagine, the device was examined by both the FDA and the manufacturer in a critical fashion with several clinical studies. Not surprisingly, both the durability and complication rate with the procedure led to the removal of this device from the market. Unfortunately, there are women that have had the Protogen placed who continue to develop problems. If you are one of these individuals, it is best to find a urologist/urogynecologist who is comfortable dealing with problems related to the use of Protogen.

85. What is the tension-free vaginal tape procedure (TVT)?

Tension free vaginal tape procedure (TVT)

type of surgical procedure in which polypropylene tape is placed under the mid-urethra, rather than at the proximal portion as with a sling procedure.

The **tension-free vaginal tape procedure (TVT)** is a fairly new procedure here in the United States. It was approved by the FDA in 1998. In Europe, more than a half million TVTs have been performed already. This procedure was developed based on the concept that stress urinary incontinence (SUI) develps when the ligaments in the middle portion of the urethra begin to

Female (midsagittal section)

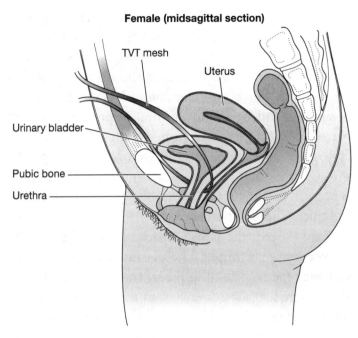

Figure 9

weaken and no longer support the urethra. Thus, this procedure is aimed at supporting the mid-urethra (see Figure 9).

The technique of the TVT procedure has some similarities to a conventional sling procedure. However, unlike the sling procedure that is placed next to the proximal urethra, the TVT is placed under the mid-urethra. In addition, the TVT material is placed under minimal to no tension. The tape is composed of a special suture-like mesh known as polypropylene and is produced by Gynecare Corporation (a division of Johnson & Johnson). An advantage of the TVT is that it may be performed under local anesthesia through a very small vaginal incision made right in the area of the mid-urethra. Special instruments known as trocars are used that pass from the vaginal incision through the pelvic floor and exit the anterior abdominal wall. The mesh tape is attached to these trocars and one trocar is placed on each slide; as the trocars are pulled up through the anterior abdominal wall, the tape is positioned under the mid-urethra. After the trocars are placed, the bladder is inspected with a cystoscope (a cystoscope is a specialized instrument that is passed through the urethra and allows one to see the inner aspect of the urethra and the bladder) to ensure that the trocars have not entered the bladder. Once the trocars are passed, the tape positioned properly, and the cystoscopy is performed, the plastic sheath is removed and the tape is secured in place. Unlike the traditional sling, there are no sutures tied to the anterior abdominal wall. Since the procedure can be performed under local anesthesia and is minimally invasive, most patients may be discharged to home within an hour or two after the procedure.

The TVT procedure has been used for over five years in the United States. Cure rates have approached 85% and improvements in urinary incontinence in up to 95% of individuals. The cure rate appears to be lower in elderly patients. The incidence of postoperative overactive bladder is low with this procedure, occurring in less than 5% of patients (see Table 7 in Question 87).

86. Who are the most appropriate patients for TVT surgery?

The TVT procedure may be utilized for women with genuine stress urinary incontinence and individuals with Type III SUI. Contraindications to a TVT procedure include women who are still considering further children and those with untreated overactive bladder. Individuals who have undergone prior renal transplant are also not candidates for a TVT procedure. Similarly, individuals who have undergone prior abdominal surgery who may have bowel adhesions are not suitable candidates for a TVT procedure.

87. What are the risks and complications associated with TVT surgery?

The risks and complications associated with TVT surgery are very low. However, as with all surgical procedures there are the risks of infection, bleeding, and pain. Other risks related to the procedure include:

Urinary retention: Urinary retention is the inability to void on your own. If this occurs, it typically is immediately after the surgery and is most often transient. Often you will be taught clean intermittent catheterization, so that you may empty your bladder without the need for an indwelling catheter. The advantage of clean intermittent catheterization is that it allows you to know when your bladder is working again (see Question 50). The general consensus is that you should be voiding on your own by eight weeks after your surgery, and that if you are not voiding on your own by this time there is an obstruction that must be treated. Usually the obstruction is due to the TVT being too tight and it resolves with releasing the TVT through another vaginal procedure.

Overactive bladder (see Question 7) occurs in 2% to 3% of patients after TVT surgery. Usually this problem is transient and can be treated with anticholinergic medications until it resolves. If the problem persists the patient may need further evaluation. Rarely, symptoms of overactive bladder may be caused by obstruction by the TVT.

Injury in the bladder and/or urethra: Injury to the bladder and/or urethra is rare. Bladder injuries include tears in the bladder or passage of the tape through the bladder. Such problems, although easy to treat when recognized, can create problems if not recognized at the time of surgery. Tears of the bladder will heal on their own, but require that a Foley catheter be left in the bladder for a week or so. Similarly, if the trocar pierces the bladder, it needs to be removed and repositioned, and then the bladder injury will heal on its own. If the tape passes through the bladder there is the risk of urinary leakage, infection, and stone formation, all of which will require additional treatment.

Deep vein thrombosis

a blood clot in the veins, usually the legs.

Deep venous thrombosis: DVT is clotting of the deep veins, and typically this occurs in the lower part of the legs during or after surgery. A DVT typically begins with leg swelling and pain in the calf of the affected leg. The DVT is treated with blood thinners to dissolve it and prevent a piece of it from passing into the heart and then the lungs, causing a pulmonary embolus, which can be fatal. The physician will give injections of a blood thinner, or place specialized stockings on the patient's legs, and/or use special hydraulic compression stockings to decrease the risk of a DVT from forming.

Death (mortality) is a complication that has been reported with the TVT procedure, but it is extremely rare. There have been seven deaths associated with the TVT procedure and six of these were associated with a

Table 7   Summary of the complications associated with TVT surgery

Complication	Rate	Number per 100,000
Vascular injury	44	9
Bowel perforation	28	6
Hematoma	20	4
Nerve injury	4	0.8

bowel injury at the time of the procedure. Although this may sound scary, it is important to take this absolute number in the context of the number of procedures being performed. This means that the mortality rate is about one to two deaths per 100,000 TVT procedures being performed.

88. How does the polypropylene mesh tape stay in place if it is not sutured in place?

There are two components that allow the tape to remain in place even though it is not secured by sutures. One component is the tape itself, which is responsible for the tape remaining in place early after surgery. The other is the healing process, which is responsible for long-term stability of the tape position. The tape itself has hair-like projections on the lateral (on the side) aspects that allow it to stick to surrounding tissue much like Velcro® sticks to cotton. This allows the tape to remain in position during the early postoperative period. The second component is the way the body heals. The tape is meshed, which means that it is woven and not completely solid. As your body heals, it lays down tissue called collagen into the mesh, and this collagen extends to the sidewalls of the pelvis. This is responsible for the improved support of the tape over the following six to eight weeks after surgery.

89. Are there any other tension-free sling procedures available for women with genuine stress urinary incontinence?

An increasing number of TVT-like procedures are being developed and marketed. Two of the most common techniques are the SPARC® sling system (manufactured by American Medical Systems, Minneapolis, MN) and the IVS Tunneller® (US Surgical and Tyco Health Care Group, Norwalk, CT).

The SPARC™ sling system uses a Prolene woven tape to provide mid-urethral support. This procedure differs from the TVT procedure in the fact that the trocars are placed through the abdominal wall down into the vaginal incision. Essentially, this is a top-down approach. Urologists are more familiar with this method of trocar placement.

The IVS Tunneller™ is a system that can be used in several different ways within the vagina. It clearly has merit in the anterior compartment (i.e., the front part of the body), which is the portion of the vagina that supports the bladder and the urethra. Here it is able to facilitate the placement of a polypropylene mesh in a tension-free fashion below the urethra to correct stress urinary incontinence. After the mesh tape is placed beneath the mid-urethra, care is taken to make sure that the tape stays flat. At that point, a device called the "delta wing" is use to move the tape up anteriorly through the lower abdominal wall. This procedure utilizes the same principles that are described in the TVT procedure (see Question 53). However, the IVS Tunneller™ system may also be used to correct what are called posterior defects, such as **rectoceles** (herniation of the anterior wall of the rectum into the vagina) as well as add support for the vaginal apex (the top of the vagina) in women who suffer from weakness of support at the top and what is called vaginal vault polapse.

Rectocele
herniation of the anterior wall of the rectum into the vagina.

90. What is the transobturator tape procedure for the treatment of SUI?

The **transobturator tape procedure** is a fairly new, minimally invasive procedure for the treatment of stress urinary incontinence. It was first developed by Mentor Corporation and started being used in the United States in 2001. It is very different than the other procedures discussed in earlier questions. Instead of trocars being placed from the adomen into the vagina or vice versa, the trocars are placed transversely across the floor of the pelvis. This allows for placement of the mesh under the urethra in a tension-free manner. The goal is to provide efficacy but less morbidity than the TVT procedure. This procedure has been modified by Johnson & Johnson Corporation in a similar but reverse manner of trocar placement. Whether one procedure is superior to the other, however, remains to be seen.

Transobturator tape procedure
a minimally invasive procedure for the treatment of stress urinary incontinence.

91. Who are appropriate candidates for the transobturator approach and what are the risks?

The candidates for tension-free sling placement via the transobturator tape approach are probably the broadest of all. If an individual meets the criteria for a sling procedure, then the transobturator tape approach would be effective. The transobturator tape approach can be used in women suffering from both genuine stress urinary incontinence and Type III stress urinary incontinence. Since the procedure is performed much deeper in the pelvis there is a much lower risk of bladder, bowel, or blood vessel injury with the transobturator approach. This procedure may be used in individuals who have undergone renal transplantation or multiple abdominal procedures, who are not good candidates for a TVT procedure.

92. Are bone anchors still used in incontinence surgery?

Given the ease of use and limited morbidity (risk of death) of anchoring screws in orthopedic surgery, researchers were enthusiastic about using bone anchors in incontinence surgery. This enthusiasm was tempered by some of the complications encountered. Since the sutures used to anchor the sling are passed through the vaginal tissue, there is the risk of infecting the bone anchor and the surrounding bone (**osteomyelitis**). The bone anchors may also cause a painful inflammation of the pubic bone, called osteitis pubis. Bone anchors may still have a role in certain individuals. People in whom bone anchors may prove helpful include those who have undergone pelvic irradiation, those who have had multiple pelvic surgeries, and those with prior chemotherapy. All of these conditions may lead to scarred and/or weakened tissues for which the bone anchor may be useful.

Osteomyelitis

inflammation of the bone marrow and adjacent bone.

PART FIVE

Physical Complications and Social Concerns of Incontinence

I'm obese. Am I a candidate for surgery?

Does natural childbirth damage the muscles for bladder control, and should I ask my obstetrician to do a cesarean section at my next delivery?

What is a prolapse?

More…

93. How do I select my urologist or urogynecologist?

Kathy's comment:

I was lucky to be working in urology. I knew many doctors in the field and it was fairly easy for me to make my decision. However, I think that you should get references from family and friends. It is also a great idea to ask nurses (if you know any) who work in the operating room (OR) with urologists. I think that a nurse can be your best identifier because she/he can evaluate skill level, etc.

Urologist

a physician who has completed a medical degree at a medical school as well as advanced training and practice in the field of urology, who is concerned with the study, diagnosis, and treatment of the genitourinary tract.

Urogynecologist

a physician who has completed a medical degree at a medical school as well as advanced training and practice in the fields of urology, who is concerned with the study, diagnosis, and treatment of the genitourinary tract, and gynecology, the study, diagnosis, and treatment of the female genital tract, as well as endocrinology and the reproductive physiology of the female.

Finding a **urologist** or **urogynecologist** to help you with your problem sometimes can be challenging. Your primary care doctor, friends, and family may be able to help you to identify potential doctors. In selecting which doctor is best for you for management of your urinary incontinence, there are several things that you may consider.

(1) Is he/she competent? Competency can be measured by answering a few questions. Is the physician board certified in this particular procedure? Board certification means that the person has completed postgraduate classes and passed a strict test of proficiency by physicians from a qualified medical school. Does the individual perform the procedure regularly such that he/she maintains his/her surgical skills? How many times has this physician performed this procedure? What are his/her success and complication rates? It is perfectly appropriate to ask such questions and the urologist/urogynecologist should be comfortable answering these questions. Make sure that you ask the doctor for his/her specific success and complication

rates. He/she may quote the results of large studies, but the doctors in the studies aren't operating on—it is the doctor that you are talking to who might perform the procedure.

(2) Do you feel comfortable with the doctor?

(3) Does your insurance company cover the procedure and the physician's costs?

94. When my doctor says that I have prolapse, what does he mean?

Kathy's comment:

Pelvic prolapse and all of its variations are described pretty well in this question. Because of my clinical background I realized that there was a common association between SUI and pelvic prolapse. However, I was under the belief that if you (the patient) had either uterine or vaginal vault pro-lapse, there would be some significant symptoms of pressure or pain that would have become bothersome somewhere along the line. Other than urine leakage, I had practically no other problems. Consequently, I was surprised when my surgeon told me that in addition to my urine leakage that I had a Grade III proplase or cystocele. To achieve the most normal postoperative result, it is best to correct the prolapse at the time of anti-incontinence surgery. Fortunately, my surgeon was able to diagnose the prolapse and fix the prob-lem at the same time as my Burch procedure.

When the doctor speaks of **prolapse**, he or she is talk-ing about the lack of support with respect to the floor and the ceiling of the vagina. This scaffolding that

Prolapse

the lack of support with respect to the floor and the ceiling of the vagina; this scaffolding that sup-ports the vagina also supports other struc-tures such as the bladder, the uterus, and the rectum.

supports the vagina also supports other structures such as the bladder, the uterus, and the rectum. At the uppermost part of the vagina is the cervix, which connects to the uterus. The rectum lies posterior (in back of) to the vagina, and the bladder and urethra lie anterior (in front of) to the vagina.

Prolapse is often divided into two categories: **uterine prolapse** and vault prolapse. **Vault prolapse** can be further categorized depending on the organ that is prolapsing and includes: bladder prolapse (cystocele), bowel prolapse (enterocele), and rectal prolapse (rectocele). Enteroceles may occur after a hysterectomy.

Prolapse is graded on a scale of 0 to IV. Grade I prolapse is mild. Grade II prolapse is descent of the vaginal wall such that it protrudes to the level of the vaginal opening, the introitus. Grade III prolapse involves descent of the vaginal wall to the introitus at rest, and descent beyond the introitus with straining. Grade IV prolapse is descent well beyond the vaginal introitus at rest.

95. Is prolapse always associated with urinary incontinence?

The answer to this question is emphatically no. However, there are a few points that are worthwhile making. With respect to stress urinary incontinence (SUI), the primary problem is a weakness or laxity of the ligaments and the soft tissue, which support the bladder and the urethra. Prolapse is really an extension of this same process. The decrease in tone allows for not only poor support of the bladder neck area, but of other areas such as the bladder base and the rectum. Therefore, if the lack of support process progresses to the point where the bladder falls, the bladder neck and the

---

Uterine prolapse

when the uterus is not supported by the pelvic floor and sinks down.

Vault prolapse

lack of support with respect to the floor and ceiling of the vagina; categorized depending on the organ that is prolapsing, including bladder prolapse (cystocele), bowel prolapse (enterocele), and rectal prolapse (rectocele). Enteroceles may occur after a hysterectomy.

urethra will not be supported. Paradoxically, if both the bladder base and the bladder neck area have fallen, the individual may not leak. However, if the bladder prolapse is corrected without supporting the bladder neck area with a sling procedure at the same time, then the patient may leak. With milder degrees of prolapse, one often sees stress urinary incontinence because of the obvious related support defects of the bladder and urethra, which allows them to fall into the potential space of the vagina and out of the realm of the normal closing pressure.

At times, prolapse can be associated with a combination of both SUI and urge urinary incontinence (UUI). The combination is referred to as mixed urinary incontinence. Occasionally, descent or prolapse of the anterior vaginal wall, which is the component that supports the bladder, can be interpreted by the patient as a sense of bladder pressure or urinary urgency. If one superimposes a stress component on this sense, the patient may experience what is known as a stress-induced involuntary bladder muscle contraction. This can cause the sense of bladder pressure and leakage as well. Therefore, although complex, prolapse may be associated with a variety of types of urinary incontinence.

96. In the patient with stress urinary incontinence associated with high-grade uterine prolapse, should a hysterectomy be done at the time of continence surgery?

Kathy's comment:

This is a common scenario for women. There is no absolute correct answer. Your decision has to depend on the experience of your surgeon in dealing with these types of problems along with your (the patient) personal feelings on having the uterus removed. When I had my laprascopic Burch procedure and cystocele repair, I did not have a hysterectomy performed. I had strong feelings about keeping my uterus, so unless there was practically no chance for me to achieve continence with my uterus in place, I was going to keep it. It has been several years since my surgery and I have no leakage problems at all.

This combination of entities, that is, stress urinary incontinence with high-grade uterine prolapse, is not commonly seen in urogynecologic circles. It is important to note that many competent physicians will treat this differently and still have good outcomes.

However, to answer this question, it must be viewed purely from the standpoint of stress urinary incontinence. This issue was examined extensively in the literature on three occasions. One study suggested that if one was preparing to perform a retropubic suspension in a patient with stress urinary incontinence and associated high-grade uterine prolapse, that voiding dynamics were improved if one performed a hysterectomy at the same sitting. However, it is important to note that subsequent reviews demonstrated no advantage with respect to outcomes of urinary symptoms and voiding dynamics when hysterectomies were performed at the same time as anti-incontinence surgery. Furthermore, it was the viewpoint of the second International Consultation on Incontinence in 2001 that hysterectomy performed at the same time as incontinence surgery does not improve the improved/dry rate with respect to surgery. Nevertheless, it is also important to note that the recurrence rate with respect to the uterine prolapse in these patients is high and ranges from 24% to 80% in various studies. Thus, the role of a hysterectomy for high-grade uterine prolapse at the time of surgery for stress urinary incontinence remains controversial. The degree of prolapse and symptoms related to the prolapse will have an impact on your physician's recommendations.

97. I'm obese, and every time I cough or laugh, I leak urine to the point where it is becoming difficult for me to socialize with friends. My primary care doctor suggested that if I don't lose significant amounts of weight, then surgery could never help me. Is this true?

This idea is not uncommon in the primary care arena, especially when counseling patients regarding urinary incontinence. From the standpoint of the ability to aggravate a situation (exacerbation), obesity may play a role in making the urinary leakage worse. However, it is not really fair or even necessarily logical to assume that extra body weight that may contribute to stress-related urine leakage, precludes the ability to achieve an adequate surgical correction. To complicate this concept even further, there are no published studies that have prospectively evaluated the influence of obesity on outcomes from surgery for stress urinary incontinence. However, there have been published chart reviews that looked at this issue from a hindsight (retrospective) standpoint. These retrospective reviews focus on body mass index (BMI) as a measure of obesity. BMI is the relationship that total body fat has with the height and weight of the patient. Normal female patients should have a BMI of less than 25.

Overweight patients have BMI levels between 25 and 30, and those who are medically obese have BMI levels greater than 30. A retrospective review of women with BMIs in the obese range compared to those in the normal range showed lower cure rates for incontinence surgery for the obese patients.

Another review looked at the results of the TVT (tension-free vaginal tape) procedure in obese and non-obese females with incontinence and found no difference between the two groups.

Thus, there are no clear data supporting the idea that obesity will have a negative impact on the cure rate of stress incontinence surgery.

98. My first child was delivered naturally. Everything went fine, but occasionally if I laugh really hard, I will leak a bit of urine. Does natural childbirth damage the muscles for bladder control and should I ask my obstetrician to do a cesarean section at my next delivery?

Kathy's comment:

I think it is important to remember that in a traumatic delivery the clinical effects may sometimes take years to develop. This is especially true when there is documented damage to the soft tissues of the pelvic floor. I had 4 children. They were all vaginal (normal is how some people refer to it) deliveries. My first child was 8 pounds, numbers

2 and 3 weighed 9 pounds, and the fourth was small at 5 pounds. With the first baby, I had a 4th-degree tear of the pelvic floor. I really had no problem with incontinence until my youngest was about 13 years old.

Urinary incontinence as well as different types of pelvic prolapse has long been considered an inevitable consequence of natural childbirth. The three most common types of prolapse encountered after childbirth are: cystocele, which is the bladder dropping; rectocele, which is the rectum herniating into the vagina; and uterine prolapse, whereby the uterus drops into the vagina. Certainly, natural childbirth is probably the most significant cause of SUI in women in the United States. However, this is magnified by the fact that the risk of developing SUI and pelvic prolapse increases with advancing age. Important questions to ask are, "How does this happen and what can be done to prevent it?"

The bladder, the uterus, and the rectum are all supported by a series of hammock-like muscles that make up the pelvic floor. An intact system of muscles, nerves, and connecting tissue are crucial for adequate support of the pelvic organs as well as the maintenance of continence. If a woman develops prolapse or SUI after natural childbirth, the inciting trauma usually begins in the second stage of labor. It is during this phase that the baby's head starts to move downward in the pelvic outlet. This can overstretch the nervous supply to the pelvic floor, and in some patients may even progress to actual tearing of the supporting muscles and connective tissue, leading to poor pelvic organ support that frequently results clinically in SUI or pelvic organ prolapse as the patient ages. Ultrasound evaluations of the bladder neck and urethra in women before and after delivery demonstrated a significant change in the elevation of the bladder neck after vaginal delivery.

The strength of the urethral closing muscle or sphincter can be assessed in a functional fashion by a test called the **urethral pressure profile (UPP).** This is usually done as part of an extensive urodynamic study. Several studies have examined the effects of pregnancy on the urethral pressure profile. These studies evaluated the UPP during pregnancy and eight weeks after delivery. A significant decrease in the urethral closing pressure, which is the ability for the muscle to close the bladder outlet, was noted after "normal" vaginal delivery.

At present, about 82% of women note symptoms of SUI during pregnancy. Unfortunately, the ability to predict the long-term persistence of these symptoms is difficult. It appears that after one vaginal delivery the risk for developing SUI within five years is in the range of 20%. However, if a patient develops clinically significant SUI within the first three months after delivery, then the risk of developing persistent SUI at five years rises dramatically to over 90%.

In conclusion, it is clear that there can be significant damage to the muscles and nerves of the pelvic floor associated with normal vaginal delivery. Currently, there are no studies that qualify and quantify the degree of postpartum pelvic floor damage after vaginal versus cesarian delivery. Consequently, we can only say this: cesarean section can decrease mechanical trauma to the pelvic floor and sphincteric musculature. However, it also carries with it some significant health risks to both mother and child that your obstetrician can explain.

Urethral pressure profile (UPP)

a type of diagnostic test to measure urethral closure function; involves a continual recording of pressure through a hole in a small catheter as it is pulled at a constant rate through a point in the bladder, through the vesical neck, and down the entire urethra.

The following recommendations can be made. Firstly, be aware of the relationships between the genesis of SUI and pelvic prolapse after vaginal delivery. Secondly, remember that good pelvic floor health habits, like regular pelvic floor muscle exercises before and after delivery, adoption of an upright birthing posture with avoidance, if possible, of forceps during delivery will help reduce pelvic floor damage during natural childbirth. Third, if you have had surgery for SUI and then become pregnant, it is appropriate to discuss cesarean section delivery with your obstetrician. Finally, adopting and maintaining a healthy lifestyle including lots of regular exercise could be the best preventative measure you can take to ensure good pelvic floor health.

99. It has been 10 years since my hysterectomy and now my bladder is falling out, which is really starting to become painful. My doctor says that it should be fixed but that he needs to do a sling procedure for incontinence at the same time. However, I am not leaking any urine, so is it wise to have both of these done at the same time?

Often women with a cystocele (descent of the bladder into the vaginal vault) will have weakened pelvic floor muscles and be at risk of SUI. If there is associated kinking of the urethra by the descent of the bladder, this may counteract the weakened pelvic floor muscles and keep the women dry. In these individuals, if the bladder was simply restored to its normal position (cystocele repair), then kinking would be resolved, and SUI would result. During your evaluation, your doctor may put his/her fingers into your vagina to push the bladder back into its normal position and then ask you to cough to see if leakage occurs. If your doctor is worried about this happening to you, then he/she may recommend a sling procedure or retropubic bladder neck suspension in addition to decrease your chances of postoperative SUI.

100. Where can I find additional information about overactive bladder and urinary incontinence?

Your local hospital may be able to provide you with information regarding nearby women's health centers, which will often contain information on overactive bladder and urinary incontinence. Other resources can be found in the Appendix that follows.

Appendix

Several Web sites can be valuable resources for additional information regarding overactive bladder and urinary incontinence. They include:

www.overactivebladder.com
www.apta.org
www.medicalconsumerguide.com
www.niddk.nih.gov/health/urology/uibcw/index.htm
www.urologychannel.com/incontinence
www.mdlinx.com/patientlinx/index.cfm
www.bladdercontrol.com
www.drugs.com
www.kegel-exercises.com
www.nlm.nih.gov/medlineplus/urinaryincontinence.htm
www.medicinenet.com/urinaryincontinenceartivle.htm
www.lifebeyondthebathroom.com

The following book may be helpful:

The Urinary Incontinence Sourcebook, by Diane K. Newman and Mary K. Dzurinko. New York, NY: McGraw-Hill Co.; 1999.

Glossary

Abscess: Collection of pus under the skin.

Acetylcholine: The neurotransmitter substance at cholinergic synapses of the nerve; after the nerve is stimulated, a chemical (neurotransmitter, ACH) that is released at the end of one nerve presynaptic cell, and bridges the synapse to stimulate or inhibit the postsynaptic cell; causes cardiac inhibition, vasodilation, and other parasympathetic effects.

Acontractile bladder: A bladder that does not contract.

Afferent pathway: Messages (nerve impulse signals) inflowing to the central nervous system (brain and spinal cord).

Alpha receptor agonists: Type of medication that causes the muscles around the urethra, the sphincter muscles, to tighten or contract; may also cause tightening of the muscles that surround arteries and thus result in high blood pressure.

Angiocatheter: A small tube that is inserted into a blood vessel and dye is injected into it, so that the surrounding blood vessels and capillaries can be visualized to determine if there is a leak.

Antimuscarinic agent: A medication that blocks the effects of the neurotransmitter acetylcholine's action on muscarinic receptors. Muscarinic receptors in the bladder are involved in the control of bladder muscle contraction.

Atrophic vaginitis: Low or absent estrogen levels before or after menopause, after hysterectomy, and oophorectomy.

Autoaugmentation: A surgical procedure in which a part of the bladder muscle, the detrusor, is removed from the bladder.

Behaviorial therapy: A group of treatments designed for educating an individual about his/her medical condition so strategies can be developed to minimize or eliminate the symptoms.

Biofeedback: Information about one or more of an individual's normally unconscious body processes is made available to the individual through a visual (see), auditory (hear), or tactile (touch) signal.

Bladder augmentation: A surgical procedure whereby the bladder is enlarged with patches of organ tissue from the colon or a synthetic substance.

Bladder denervation: Techniques to deaden or eliminate the nerves in the urethra, bladder, or rectum in an effort to interrupt the nerve supply to the bladder and stop bladder contractions.

Bladder outlet: Area where the bladder joins the urethra.

Blood brain barrier (BBB): Semipermeable network of the tiniest blood vessels called capillaries with special endothelial cells surrounding the brain; the barrier prevents a variety of agents such as medications from passing through and entering the brain. Its function is to protect the brain from potentially harmful substances (like certain medications), other neurotransmitters, and hormones in the body, and to maintain the brain in a constant environment.

Botulinum neurotoxin: One of the most poisonous biologic chemicals known; produced by the bacterium *Clostridium botulinum;* very small amounts can lead to paralysis.

Burch procedure: Type of surgery similar to the Marshall Marchetti and Krantz procedure, except that the pubic bone is not used to support the bladder and bladder neck; rather the sutures are placed in some strong tissue a little more lateral, in the Cooper's ligament.

Capsaicin: The active ingredient found in chili peppers; inserted directly into the bladder to overstimulate the afferent nerves, and thus decrease bladder activity until the nerves regenerate neurotransmitters.

Catheter: A tubular instrument especially designed to be passed through the urethra into the bladder to drain the bladder.

Central nervous system: Found in the brain and spinal cord; responsible for starting or preventing urination.

Chronic obstructive pulmonary disease (COPD): General term used for diseases with permanent or temporary narrowing of small bronchi in the lungs.

Clean intermittent catheterization: A type of temporary catheter to remove urine from the body on a regular basis throughout the day; usually self-accomplished by inserting the tube through the urethra to empty the bladder. Most people are able to learn the procedure; it involves learning the location of urological landmarks and the ability to reach the urethra and manipulate the equipment.

Cognition: General term encompassing thinking, learning, and memory.

Compliance: The consistency and accuracy with which a patient follows the regimen prescribed by a physician or other health care professional.

Congenital: Existing at birth; refers to physical traits, conditions, diseases, anomalies, or malformations, etc., which may be either hereditary or because of an influence occurring during gestation up to the moment of birth.

Continence: Ability to retain urine and/or feces until a proper time for their discharge.

Cystocele: Hernia-like disorder in women that occurs when the wall between the bladder and the vagina weakens and the bladder drops into the vagina.

Cystogram: A type of test where fluid called contrast material is inserted through a catheter placed into the bladder and x-rays are obtained. The contrast material causes specific areas of the body to be "lit up" by the x-rays, so that the radiologist can analyze the area.

Cystometrogram (CMG): A component of the urodynamic study when the bladder is being filled and the pressures within the bladder are being measured.

Cystoscope: A long telescope-like instrument that is passed through the urethra into the bladder for diagnostic and therapeutic purposes. It allows one to visualize inside the bladder and urethra.

Cystoscopy: A procedure in which the bladder and urethra are examined through a narrow telescope-like

device that is passed through the urethra into the bladder.

Darifenacin (Enablex, Novartis): An antimuscarinic agent that is selective for the M3 receptor, the one responsible for bladder contractility in the normal bladder.

Deep vein thrombosis (DVT): A blood clot in the veins, usually the legs.

Detrusor: The bladder muscle. Coordinated contraction of the detrusor and opening of the bladder outlet allows for normal urination.

Diverticula: Pouch or sac outpouching from a tubular or saccular organ such as the gut or bladder.

Duloxetine: A type of medication for stress urinary incontinence that is not yet approved by the FDA. Side effect: nausea.

Efferent pathway: Messages (nerve impulse signals) outflowing from the central nervous system to the peripheral nervous system.

Efficacy: Extent to which a specific intervention, procedure, regimen, or service produces a beneficial result under ideal conditions.

Electromyography: Type of noninvasive test using skin patches to measure the activity in muscles.

Embolism: Obstruction or occlusion of a vessel.

Enterocystoplasty: A surgical procedure to enlarge the bladder by the addition of a segment of small or large intestine.

Erosion: When the pubovaginal sling migrates from its position between the urethra and the vagina and relocates in one of the two organs.

Estrogens: A class of drugs, orally or topically applied, which may be used by urologists and urogynecologists to make the urethral tissue healthier.

Fascia: A sheet of connective tissue covering or binding together body structures.

Fistula: A communication between two organs; for example, a vesicovaginal fistula, whereby the bladder and vagina are connected by a small, open tract that allows urine to pass from the bladder into the vagina.

Fluoroscopy: Visualization of tissues and deep structures of the body by x-ray.

Frequency volume chart: A document plotting the amount of urine, and number of times an individual urinates over a period of time.

Functional incontinence: A situation in which the bladder, urethra, and pelvic floor muscles are functioning properly, but physical or mental function interferes with one's ability to independently get to the bathroom on time.

Gastrocystoplasty: Similar to enterocystoplasty, except that instead of using a piece of intestine, a segment of the stomach is used to patch the bladder.

Hematoma: A collection of blood that forms in a tissue, organ, or body space as a result of a broken blood vessel.

Hypertension: Transitory or sustained elevated arterial blood pressure. Untreated, it can cause cardiovascular damage.

Imipramine: An antidepressant medication used for overactive bladder; it has antimuscarinic properties and acts on two neurotransmitters in the brain (serotonin and noradrenaline) involved in the complex interactions related to normal bladder filling and emptying.

Incision: A cut, a surgical wound.

Ingelman-Sundberg procedure: A transvaginal surgical technique that denerves the bladder to achieve control over uninhibited bladder contractions.

In-situ vaginal wall sling: Type of incontinence surgery that uses a segment of the patient's own vaginal wall to act as a hammock to support the bladder.

Intravesical: Medication placed directly into the bladder.

Kegel exercises: Exercises designed to strengthen weak pelvic floor muscles.

Kelly procedure: A surgical procedure usually performed in conjunction with a vaginal or "partial" hysterectomy in patients who have a combination of uterine descent and urinary leakage.

Laparoscopy: A minimally invasive surgical procedure that allows a view of the entire contents of the abdomen through the use of a specialized instrument, which is attached to a light source, fiberoptic camera, and surgical tools that are passed through small incisions under the umbilicus (belly button) and at other sites on the abdomen.

Local anesthesia: A short-acting spinal anesthetic or intravenous sedation.

Lower urinary tract symptoms (LUTS): Term used to describe obstructive and irratative voiding symptoms.

Marshall Marchetti and Krantz procedure (MMK): A type of surgical procedure where sutures are placed in the tissue surrounding the urethra and tacked behind the pubic bone, hence the term retropubic; the sutures are placed to provide support to the bladder and bladder neck/ proximal urethra so that increases in abdominal pressure will be transmitted to both the bladder and the proximal urethra.

Micturition: The action of voiding urine.

Mixed urinary incontinence: Involuntary leakage of urine associated with urgency as well as with exertion, effort, sneezing, or coughing. The combination of urge incontinence and stress urinary incontinence.

Mucosa: A mucous tissue lining various tubular structures, including the bladder.

Mucosal anesthesia: A type of procedure still being studied where an anesthetic agent is placed into the urethra, bladder, or rectum, to affect the sensory fibers in the bladder. In theory, if the patient responds to this procedure, it would confirm that the problem is one of bladder sensation stimulating the overactivity.

Muscarinic receptor: A membrane-bound protein that contains a recognition site for acetylcholine; combination of acetylcholine with the receptor initiates a physiologic change (i.e., slowing of the heart rate, increased glandular activity, and stimulation of smooth muscle contractions).

Neuromodulation: Surgical placement of a permanent continuous nerve stimulator and its electrode wires.

Nocturia: Having to wake from sleep at night to urinate after a day of normal fluid intake; causes include increased urine production at night, incomplete bladder emptying, sleep problems, or overactive bladder.

Obstruction: Outflow of urine from the bladder is blocked; may be caused by prostate enlargement or urethral strictures, narrowed areas in the urethra, or medications that affect the function of the urethra, among others.

Open abdominal procedures for SUI: Surgical procedures performed through an abdominal incision; used to treat SUI; typically referred to as "retropubic bladder neck suspensions" or more commonly, bladder suspensions.

Orthostatic hypotension: Lowering of blood pressure while moving from a sitting to a standing position; potential for dizziness and collapsing.

Osteitis pubis: Pain above the pubic bone that may radiate to the thighs and is made worse by walking or spreading the legs. There is often tenderness to touch over the pubic bone.

Osteomyelitis: Inflammation of the bone marrow and adjacent bone.

Overactive bladder: A symptom complex characterized by urgency, often associated with urinary frequency and nocturia, may be associated with age incontinence. Suggestive of underlying uninhibited detrosor muscle contractions.

Oxybutynin: One of the oldest pharmaceutical therapies for overactive bladder. It is effective, but its use is limited by a high incidence of side effects, including dry mouth and constipation.

Oxybutynin extended release (Ditropan XL, J&J): A type of pharmaceutical therapy for overactive bladder. It is similar to oxybutynin, but is a sustained release formulation with less dry mouth and constipation than oxybutynin.

Pelvic floor muscles: A series of muscles that form a sling or hammock across the outlet of the pelvis; these muscles, together with their surrounding tissue, are responsible for keeping all of the pelvic organs (bladder, uterus, and rectum) in place and functioning correctly.

Pelvic inflammatory disease (PID): Acute or chronic pus-forming inflammation of female pelvic structures due to infection by *Neisseria gonorrhoeae*, *Chlamydia trachomatis*, and other sexually transmitted diseases.

Pelvic prolapse: A weakening in the pelvic floor muscles that allows organs to descend out of the pelvis.

Perineum: Area between the thighs extending from the tail bone (coccyx) to the pubis (between the vulva and anus in the female and scrotum and anus in the male) and lying below the pelvic diaphragm.

Peripheral nervous system: Nerves connecting in the body other than the brain and spinal cord; responsible for the coordination of bladder contraction and urethral relaxation during normal voiding.

Periurethral injection: A type of shot where a needle filled with the agent to be injected is inserted alongside the urethra and the material injected. May be used in the treatment of Type III SUI.

Poor contractility: Where the bladder muscle cannot generate and/or sustain a contraction that completely empties it of urine; may result from damage to the nerves supplying the bladder (spinal cord injury or conditions like spina bifida), chronic overdistention of the bladder, severe long-term blockages of the outlet, or medications.

Poorly compliant bladder: Holds urine at higher than normal bladder pressures, causing poor emptying of the kidneys, a backup of urine in the kidneys, and eventually kidney damage.

Postprostatectomy urinary incontinence: Leakage of urine in men who have had a radical prostatectomy; in most cases, this resolves after the pelvic muscles heal.

Postvoid residual urine: The amount of urine left in the bladder after voiding; if elevated may lead to urinary tract infections, bladder stones, further distention of the bladder, worsening of bladder function, or dilation of the kidneys and ureter.

Potty training: Ability of toddlers to learn how to hold their urine and then voluntarily empty the bladder at a socially acceptable time. The process involves maturity as the brain develops a communication network with the bladder.

Pressure flow study: A specialized study used to assess whether there is any obstruction to the outflow of urine.

Probanthine bromide: A nonselective antimuscarinic medication for overactive bladder; individual doses will vary.

Prolapse: The lack of support with respect to the floor and the ceiling of the vagina; this scaffolding that supports the vagina also supports other structures such as the bladder, the uterus, and the rectum. If these organs are not well supported, they may descend/herniate into the vagina.

Pubovaginal sling: Type of surgical procedure that uses a synthetic or fascial sling that is placed under the proximal urethra to support the bladder neck and proximal urethra.

Radical prostatectomy: A procedure performed for prostate cancer. Includes removal of the prostate, seminal vesicles, and part of the vas deferens.

Radiofrequency: A form of electromagnetic energy that is almost a generic term for electricity.

Rectocele: Herniation of the anterior wall of the rectum into the vagina.

Resiniferatoxin: A chemical derived from a cactus-like plant, *Euphorbia resinifera*; inserted directly into the bladder to overstimulate the afferent nerves, and thereby decrease bladder activity until the nerves regenerate neurotransmitters.

Sacrum: Refers to the large, irregular, triangular shaped bone made up of the five fused vertebrae below the lumbar region; comprises part of the pelvis.

Skin patch electrodes: A noninvasive, no-pain method used in testing muscle activity or pressures involving a flat adhesive patch with embedded wires.

Small capacity bladder: Organ cannot hold much urine because of fibrosis or scarring or neurologic causes; the bladder loses its elasticity so the individual must urinate more frequently.

Solifenacin: (Vesicare, Yamanouchi) An antimuscarinic medication recently approved by the FDA for use in overactive bladder.

Sphincter mechanism: The muscular mechanism that helps maintain continence.

Stasis: When there is high pressure in the bladder, the ureter is unable to push the urine into the bladder, causing a backup of urine within the ureter and eventually the kidneys.

Stress urinary incontinence: (also known as genuine stress urinary incontinence, GSUI) Involuntary loss of bladder control during periods of increased abdominal pressure such as coughing, laughing, heavy lifting, or straining.

Suprapubic tube: A type of tube placed directly into the bladder at the time of surgery, that exits through the skin on your lower abdomen to drain the bladder; less irritating than a Foley catheter.

Tension-free vaginal tape (TVT) procedure: Type of surgical procedure where polypropylene tape is placed under the mid-urethra, rather than at the proximal portion as with a sling procedure. The TVT material is placed under minimal to no tension. An advantage of the TVT is that it may be performed under local anesthesia through a very small vaginal incision made right in the area of the mid-urethra.

Timed voiding: A type of therapy that involves urinating at two- to three-hour intervals, no matter if there is an urge.

Tissue engineering: A pioneering technique of growing cells designed to mimic the behavior and reproducibility of normal cells.

Tolterodine: First antimuscarinic drug that was developed solely for use in overactive bladder.

Tolterodine, Pfizer (Detrol LA): Type of antimuscarinic drug developed in a capsule containing small microspheres that are released slowly into the body, allowing for a sustained release of medication; used for overactive bladder and has a lower incidence of side effects.

Transcutaneous: Denotes the passage of substances through the unbroken skin.

Transdermal: Medication is delivered to the body by a skin patch.

Transdermal oxybutynin (Oxytrol, Watson): A patch formulation of oxybutynin that is changed twice a week. The patch delivers 3.9 mg of oxybutynin per day.

Transient incontinence: Leakage of urine caused by illness or medications that increase the volume of urine produced to the point where it interferes with normal urinary tract function and affects normal bladder function.

Transobturator procedure: A minimally invasive procedure for the treatment of stress urinary incontinence.

Transurethral injection: A type of shot where a cystoscope is inserted into the urethra and a thin, long needle is advanced through the cystoscope, into the urethra; the chemical is then injected into the urethra to treat Type III SUI.

Transurethral prostatectomy: Removal of the prostate through the urethra.

Transvaginal needle suspension: A type of surgical procedure used to correct SUI in the 1950s–1980s. Commonly performed procedures included the Pereyra procedure, the Stamey procedure, the Raz procedure, and the Gittes procedure.

Tricyclic antidepressants: A class of medications which may be used to treat incontinence. They lower the bladder pressure by relaxing the bladder muscle and also help further by tightening the sphincter muscle.

Trocar: In incontinence procedures, it is a specialized instrument that may be passed from the abdomen into the vagina (or vice versa) to allow for placement of a sling or suture for a transvaginal needle suspension.

Trospium chloride (Sanctura, Inderus): An antimuscarinic medication for overactive bladder that has been recently approved for use in the United States by the FDA; it is unlikely to penetrate the brain and thus does not appear to affect cognitive function.

Type III stress incontinence: Where the urethra itself doesn't close, so any increase in bladder pressure overpowers the urethra and causes leakage of urine.

Ultrasound: A noninvasive test using radiowaves (frequency greater than 30,000 MHz); used to evaluate the kidneys and bladder to assess bladder emptying capacity.

Ureter: A long, thin, hollow tubular structure connecting the kidneys to the bladder. It propels urine from the kidneys into the bladder.

Ureterocystoplasty: Technique is used in patients who have a dilated distal ureter, which can be isolated, opened, and used as a bladder patch.

Urethra: Canal leading from the bladder to the body's skin to discharge urine externally. In the female, it is ~4 cm long and opens in the perineum between the clitoris and vaginal opening; in the male it is ~20 cm long and opens in the glans penis.

Urethral pressure profile (UPP): A type of diagnostic test to measure urethral closure function; involves a continual recording of pressure through a hole in a small catheter as it is pulled at a constant rate through a point in the bladder, through the vesical neck, and down the entire urethra.

Urethral resistance profile (URP): Measurement used in urodynamic studies to determine the strength of the urethra.

Urethral sphincter: A muscle that when contracted closes the urethra.

Urge incontinence: Unintended leakage or loss of urine into clothing or bedclothes as a result of an uninhibited detrusor contraction.

Urinalysis: A type of test of the urine to determine normalcy or abnormality.

Urinary frequency: Having to void more than eight times per day with normal intake of fluids.

Urinary incontinence: Involuntary loss of urine. May be the result of an overactive bladder, stress incontinence, functional incontinence, or other causes.

Urinary retention: The inability to urinate on one's own.

Urinary urgency: Sudden compelling desire to urinate that often is difficult to defer.

Urine cytology: A small amount of urine is sent to the pathologist, who examines the urine sample to determine the presence or absence of any cancer cells.

Urodynamic study: A special test used to determine how the bladder and urethral muscles work; includes measuring storage and emptying of the bladder.

Uroflow: The rate of flow of the urine stream; often a component of a urodynamic study, but may be performed in the office.

Urogynecologist: A specialty trained physician who has completed a medical degree at a medical school as well as advanced training and practice in the fields of urology, who is concerned with the study, diagnosis, and treatment of the genitourinary tract, and gynecology, the study, diagnosis, and treatment of the female genital tract, as well as endocrinology and the reproductive physiology of the female.

Urologist: A physician who has completed a medical degree at a medical school as well as advanced training and practice in the field of urology, who is concerned with the study, diagnosis, and treatment of the genitourinary tract.

Urothelium: Type of cell that lines the urinary tract.

Uterine prolapse: When the uterus is not supported by the pelvic floor and sinks down.

Valsalva leak point pressure: The intra-abdominal pressure generated by a Valsalva maneuver that results in urinary leakage.

Valsalva maneuver: Any forced expiratory effort ("strain") against a closed airway; used to study cardiovascular effects as well as poststrain responses.

Vault prolapse: Lack of support with respect to the floor and ceiling of the vagina; categorized depending on the organ that is prolapsing, including bladder prolapse (cystocele), bowel prolapse (enterocele), and rectal prolapse (rectocele). Enteroceles may occur after a hysterectomy.

Vesicoureteral reflux: Urine passing backwards from the bladder to the kidneys.

Videourodynamics: Use of intermittent fluoroscopy (taking x-ray pictures) during the urodynamic study to visualize the bladder and urethra.

Void: To evacuate urine and/or feces.

Warning time: Duration of time between the individual's initial perception of urinary urgency and the onset of voiding or incontinence.

Xenografts: Biologic tissues that are removed from other species and used in human transplantation.

Index